MORNING SICKNESS

HOW YOU CAN HAVE A NAUSEA-FREE PREGNANCY WITH THESE NEW RAW FOOD SECRETS AND NATURAL REMEDIES

PATRICIA DE KUIPER, MSC

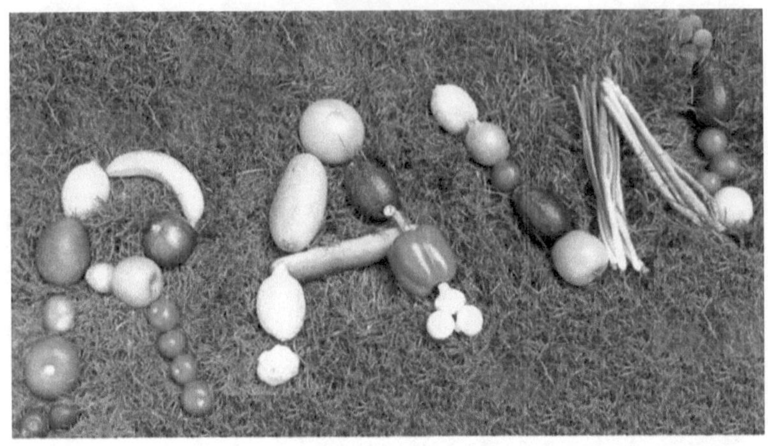

HOW TO HAVE A NAUSEA-FREE PREGNANCY WITH THESE NEW RAW FOOD SECRETS AND NATURAL REMEDIES

Patricia de Kuiper, MSc

I dedicate this book to my childen, who inspired me to take the next step in healing through nutrition

Spacepat publishing

www.spacepat.com

Kindle ISBN: 97 81 73 13 18 572

Disclaimer:

The contents of this book such as text, graphics, images and other material contained in this book are for informational purposes only. The content is not intended to be a substitute for professional medical advice, diagnosis, or treatment. Always seek the advice of your physician or other qualified health provider with any questions you may have regarding a medical condition. Never disregard professional medical advice or delay in seeking it because of something you have read in this book.

If you think you have a medical emergency, call your doctor or you local emergency service immediately. This book shares personal experience only and does not recommend or endorse any specific tests, physicians, products, procedures, opinions or other information that may be mentioned in this book. Reliance on any information provided by this books solely at your own risk.

This book may contain health- or medical-related material that is sexually explicit. If you find these materials offensive, you may not want to read this book.

Contents

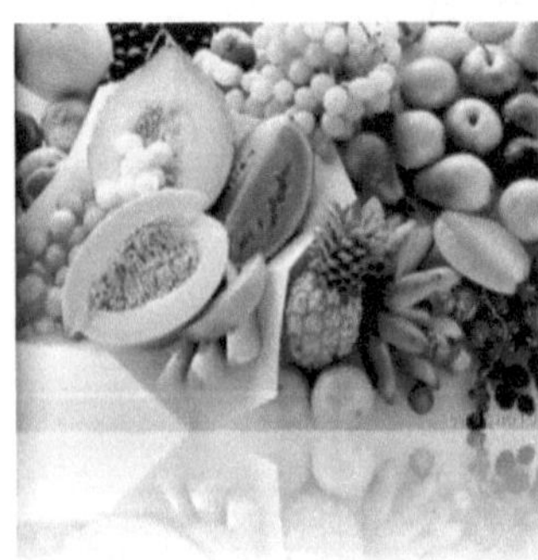

My Story

We had been trying for six years and I had become used to and expectant of the "not pregnant" verdict.
The first time I received the news that I was pregnant, I couldn't believe it. It felt like this news wasn't meant for me but for somebody else.

After it sunk in, I was surprised about the depth of the joy I was feeling. It seemed like a physical happiness, not coming from the mind but coming from within every cell of my body. Greater and shinier than anything I had ever felt before. I didn't know happiness like that even existed, let alone that I could ever experience it myself! I felt so grateful!

It didn't take very long though for me to start to feel nauseous. Strangely enough, the feeling of nausea made me happy too! It acted as a constant reminder, confirming my pregnancy. At the same time, the feeling of nausea was very intense and overwhelming. It was tiring, unpractical and debilitating. I had no idea how to cope with it. At the same time my nausea developed, my body started rejecting all foods that were not Raw. Meaning, I only could eat raw fruits, vegetables, nuts and seeds. Chocolate, french fries, bread, meat, diary, things I had loved before, it all tasted dead and repulsive to me. My body simply forced me into a Raw Vegan diet. However even though raw vegan food seemed to help my body feel better, it didn't completely stop me from feeling the nausea.

One day, I was walking downtown and came across a brand new juice store that sold wheatgrass juice. I had tried wheatgrass juice in the past but my juicer at the time was not able to juice wheatgrass so I was very happy to be able to buy it. I did not like the taste of the wheatgrass juice. Most probably, I wasn't the only one who did not find the juice delectable because the juice shop offered a free shot of pineapple juice to wash away the taste! Unfortunately the taste remained, but to my amazement, after having the juice, my nausea disappeared like snow in the sun. What an amazingly easy solution!

My skeptical self wondered if it was truly because of the wheatgrass juice. Now I had a reason to worry. I never really thought whether it is safe to drink wheatgrass juice while pregnant. But I also realised that my feelings of nausea had vanished that day. I went back and tried the juice again and found that the days I drank wheatgrass juice, I had no nausea! So, this became a regular routine through my pregnancy. As I drank the juice, I came across other solutions as well. I tried several of these natural foods.

I guess the raw food and the wheatgrass juice worked on other levels too: my doctor kept telling me through my pregnancy that my blood tests were super healthy. My iron levels were excellent, which is usually a concern during pregnancy. And when my baby was three weeks old, the doctor said that she had never seen such a strong baby! In fact, she was amazed at how quickly my baby could up her head.

That wasn't all. My endocrinologist told me that the thyroid problem I had been struggling with had diminished as well! You can imagine how grateful I was that I discovered the raw foods that helped me through my pregnancy.

After my pregnancy, I started researching about pregnancy nausea and natural remedies for it. I came across so much information that at times it was almost impossible to sift the wheat from the chaff. But I didn't give up. I continued to research and experiment with a passion.

Through my research I read accounts of several hundred women, during and after their pregnancy. What I discovered was that women who were on a raw food diet through their pregnancy unanimously reported positive effects, including excellent blood levels, good iron levels and healthy babies. They said that their babies were aware and alert and made eye contact very early on. As compared to women who did not include raw foods in their diet through pregnancy, women on a raw diet also report easier deliveries, with some even saying that their delivery was not only faster but also painless. The fact is that not a single woman on a raw diet reported a lack of benefits from their food plan. They also said that they did not experience the usual pregnancy symptoms, such as water retention.

This research led me to not only come up with a list of raw foods that offer the most benefits during pregnancy but it also gave me the motivation to write a book on raw pregnancy that could help women all over the world. I also launched a website, www.rawpregnancy.com, to ensure that every woman feels at their best during pregnancy. The website has been ranked Number #1 on Google, the most popular search engine. Apart from this, I am active on various popular social networking sites and own several online raw pregnancy communities.

I am not a medical practitioner, nor do I have any medical training. I'm not a midwife not a dietician either. The information and recommendations included in this book are based my personal experiences and on the 20 long years I have spent exploring and researching facts on food philosophies, raw foods and how they help overcome pregnancy related nausea. There is no one ultimate solution and nor do I claim that I have all the answers. These are practical recommendations from many different women, based on experience and on their proven effectiveness that I have gathered through my research.

I believe that a raw pregnancy is the greatest gift you can give to your child. I also understand that different women experience pregnancy differently. Through my book, Morning Sickness, I hope to address the common experience of pregnancy nausea and suggest ways to overcome this nausea in a healthy way.

To help you come up with a customized solution for your specific needs, this book discusses:

- Choice of the right raw foods: Firstly, the reader will get to know about specific raw foods that can make a dramatic difference in whether a pregnant woman feels nausea or not. There are specific raw foods and raw superfoods that have helped pregnant women fight morning sickness. Even when there is minimal or no nausea, these foods can prove beneficial during pregnancy.

- Optimizing the intake of selected raw food solutions: Pregnant women need to choose specific raw food solutions and optimize their intake to ensure maximum positive effect. I would recommend that you not only take notes while reading this book but keep a record of when you feel nauseous. This will help you understand your symptoms and experience better and therefore identify effective solutions.

- Appropriate system for specific pregnancy situation: According to the situation of your pregnancy and depending on the test results, this book will guide you on how to select a solution that works best for you. It is important that the solution is tailor-made to the needs of each individual for the person to gain the maximum benefits.

So, get ready to enjoy this period of your life by arming yourself with the right information.

What Is Morning Sickness

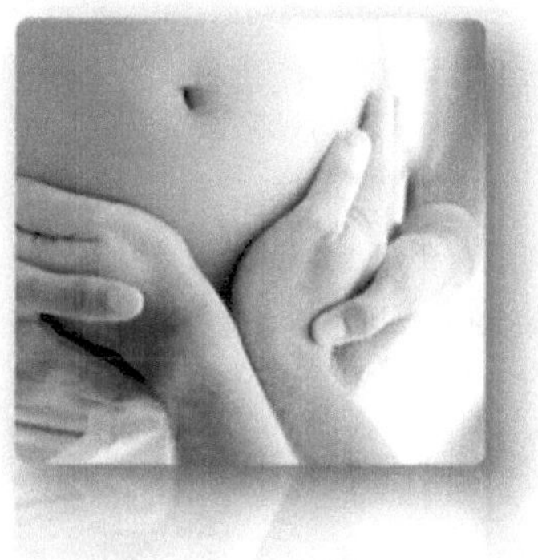

Morning sickness can be listed among the worst things a woman experiences in her entire life. The nausea can be so intense and long-lasting, that it can drive women to the limits of despair.

Meanwhile, the medical profession does not always appreciate the seriousness of this problem. Doctors sometimes feel that it is a healthy expression of the fact that there is a pregnancy. Even worse, they can be belittling and degrading to women who try to get their help, and feel that these women should not complain about this minor, even cute, side effect of their pregnancy.

Pregnancy nausea can drive women, who want their baby more than anything in the world, to such despair that they actually get an abortion to end their nausea ordeal. Some women are no longer able to eat because they just vomit out everything they consume.

Strangely, babies of women who have experienced nausea during their pregnancy statistically end up being healthier than babies whose mother didn't feel nauseous at all during pregnancy.

At the same time, most doctors who will take their patients seriously simply have no real medical answers to help with the nausea. That is where simply sharing experiences becomes helpful. Have you found something that actually works for you? Please join our community and share it at http://rawpregnancy.com/community. The solutions in this book came from women sharing what has really worked for them and from further reasoning of what similar solutions might also work.

The term "Morning Sickness" is really a misnomer. Most women who have ever experienced it can tell you that it isn't only in the morning that you feel nauseous. In medical terms, "Nausea and Vomiting of Pregnancy" (NVP) is used to describe morning sickness. Judicious choice of words makes it clear that a pregnant woman can feel nauseous at any time of the day and this feeling need not be limited to a particular time of the day. On the other hand, not everyone who is pregnant feels nauseous.

From my personal experience, I agree that "Morning sickness" is not the appropriate term. However everybody uses this term and everybody knows what you mean. It is like a folklore term and we'll just keep using it.

Most pregnant women feel nauseous during the initial stages of their pregnancy, after they wake up in the morning; mostly several weeks into the first trimester. Some women do not feel nauseous at all, some feel so in the mornings and then there are many pregnant women who feel nauseous for the entire day, throughout the pregnancy. However, the intensity may vary from one moment to another.

Nausea can lead to disruption in one's normal lifestyle, missed work, disturbance in sleep, fatigue and irritability. On a macro level, nausea can have a significant socio-economic repercussion due to the hours lost in paid employment.

Emotional stress, travel, and the smell or taste of some foods can aggravate such feelings.

Morning Sickness - The Symptoms

So just to summarise, the most common symptoms of morning sickness
include:

1. Sickness
2. Nausea
3. Vomiting
4. Dislike for some foods
5. Loss of appetite
6. Psychological effects, such as depression and anxiety

The way these symptoms work out can be very different. The nausea can last all
day, or it can come in waves. In my second pregnancy, I experienced very acute
nausea every time I entered a room that was not heated well, or sometimes
when I smelled something my body apparently didn't like, or simply when I was
tired after a long day. I only vomited if I would fail to take care of the
circumstances, like if I would not get warm, get out of the smelly space or rest. I
am sure your symptoms are slightly different from the ones you hear from other
women. It's just very different from person to person.

Morning Sickness - The Causes

Up to this day, science has never been able to pinpoint one specific cause of pregnancy nausea. Some of the possible causes of pregnancy nausea could be:

1. Hormonal changes – The hormones, Human chorionic gonadotropin (hCG) and Estrogen, rise rapidly during pregnancy. There are continuous changes at the hormonal level. During the course of pregnancy, the placenta develops and releases pregnancy hormones, including HCG, estrogen and progesterone, disrupting the internal balance of pregnant women. The presence of hCG is associated with morning sickness, so much so that after a miscarriage, this hormone takes a couple weeks to disappear from your blood, and can still cause feelings of nausea.
2. Sensitivity to smell or odours – Probably due to hormonal changes.
3. The gastrointestinal tract in some people becomes more sensitive to changes that occur during early pregnancy. As a result, the probability to gastric reflux, nausea and vomiting increases, despite maintaining a healthy and balanced diet. This may be the result of evolution: those mothers who were more careful of what they ate had better chances for survival and this aspect of evolution led to a supersensitivity in some pregnant women.
4. Lack of nourishment: vitamins, minerals, etc. For example, lack of vitamin B6 may lead to hyperemesis gravidarum, a severe form of nausea and vomiting in pregnancy. The body becomes extra sensitive to insufficient nourishment because the new baby needs everything in the right amount to be able to grow.
5. Fluctuations in blood pressure. The amount of blood in the body increases because the mother's blood goes through the new baby's body. This may cause some adaptation problems in the form of varying blood pressure.
6. Changes in metabolism that occur during pregnancy, for example the carbohydrate metabolism changes

7. Insufficient nutrition. It is my personal conviction that poor quality nutrition may not just be at the root of pregnancy nausea, but at the root of most chronic conditions.

8. Toxicity. Not even a hundred years ago, all food was organic. Nowadays there is toxicity everywhere. Pesticides, food preservatives, artificial food colouring, car emissions, industrial emissions, magnetic fields, radiation, the list goes on. Cancer used to be a rare disease but nowadays it kills one in three people. Even though the food industry and government tells us that we are within safe limits, should we believe that? the toxins build up in our bodies, our livers get overburdened and it it my personal belief that our bodies simply are too overburdened to be able to deal with the extra demands that pregnancy puts on out body.

Since there are so many different solutions for pregnancy nausea, it would be plausible that there are different causes.

I believe that the first step in coping with pregnancy nausea is to either try out the different solutions found in this book or reason which cause is more likely and then try that solution first. This way you might find cures that will work at the very root of the problem. We will discover these solutions through the course of this book.

Why Should We Seek Solutions for Morning Sickness?

There are written accounts of nausea and vomiting during pregnancy from as early as 2,000 BC and the Ancient Egyptians didn't seem to have found the best cure for this condition either.

Statistics tell us that 85% of all pregnant women experience some form of morning sickness or pregnancy-related nausea. The degree to which they experience nausea does, however, differ from one person to another, with some women experiencing the most severe morning sickness, known as Hyperemesis Gravidarum. Again, statistics tell us that one in every 300 pregnant women experience this severe condition. A woman with Hyperemesis Gravidarum could even end up weighing 5% less that she did before she got pregnant!

What is worrying about morning sickness is that it can take a toll on your health. Although morning sickness itself does not directly affect the baby, if the expectant mother is malnourished or dehydrated due to pregnancy nausea, or affected psychologically, then these conditions are simply very undesirable. This only suggests that seeking solutions for morning sickness is very important. Various medical and non-medical remedies have been tried over the years by women all over the world. While there is no single best remedy, some remedies are extremely effective for some women, while others find relief in different types of solutions.

Treat Yourself Effectively with Life Style Changes, Raw Vegan Food and Natural Remedies

This brings me to the main theme of this book – natural solutions and raw foods. I have tried several solutions and their effectiveness blew me away. I believe they even helped my unborn baby, nourishing her to make her so strong and healthy that my Caregiver was just amazed at her strength.

Life Style and Home Remedies For Morning Sickness

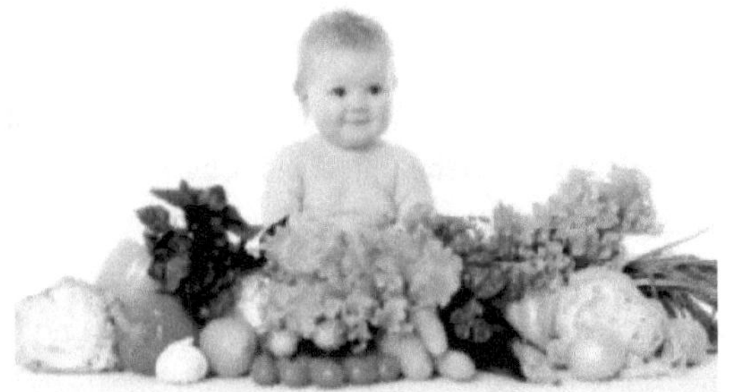

1 *Eat small meals, frequently.*

Most people working with pregnant women suggest that women experiencing pregnancy nausea should eat about five or six times a day. They should ensure that these are small meals that do not add too much bulk to the stomach at one time. This is because both hunger pangs and a feeling of being overfull can trigger nausea. When we are hungry, the acids in the stomach have no food to digest and therefore cause discomfort, while eating a large meal causes a feeling of being too full for the stomach to handle quickly.

2 *Drink fluids*

Your stomach might find it easier to deal with liquids rather than solids when you are nauseous. Soups, juices and other fluids can help you feel better. Keep yourself well hydrated to take the edge off morning sickness. Ensure you take more fluids, even water with a slice of lemon, during this time.
Dehydration can cause morning sickness. It always nice to drink water for multiple benefits such as cleansing the digestive system and staying hydrated enough to prevent loss of excess body water.

3 *Avoid heavy spices*

Spicy foods could aggravate nausea. Stay with foods that have a natural flavor that you like and avoid foods containing too many spices.

4 *Drink lots of water*

Making sore that you are sufficiently hydrated may prevent morning sickness caused by unconscious dehydration. Something as simple as drinking more water may be the answer for you! Sweetened water works too. Water before and after meals has also been found to reduce the experience of nausea.

5 *Crackers*

Crackers like chips, have been found to alleviate morning sickness. Especially when eaten in bed before you get up in the morning. Have them next to your bed so you can eat some immediately after waking up. You may use healthier alternatives like Raw Kale Crisps or Chia seed crackers.

6 *Get your daily dose of vitamins and minerals*

During pregnancy, it is vital that you ensure the intake of the necessary vitamins and minerals, such as Vitamin B6 and folic acid. Malnutrition is one of the causes of morning sickness. Off course it is important to not overdo this and stick to daily recommended amounts. Raw foods like green juices may go a long way in taking care of your nutritional needs in a more healthy way.

7 *Walk every day*

Walking is a low impact exercise that not only helps you feel better, it can alleviate nausea and as a bonus helps to prepare you for birth-giving.

8 *Start slow and avoid sudden moves*

Start your day slowly. You are pregnant. Relax and enjoy the experience rather than rushing around from the time you wake up. Keep your morning activities slow and calm. Also avoid making sudden posture changes when you get out of bed or out of a chair.

9 *Get enough sleep*

I cannot over emphasise the importance of sleep. Unfortunately, this is also one aspect that most of us underestimate in terms of its effect on the body.

While these solutions may work for many, enough times I have heard from women who have more or less tried all of these and nothing worked. Since they are very gentle there's no harm in trying them, you might as well start out by give each of them a try. However if they do not work then try the other solutions offered later in this book.

10 *Acupressure Wristbands*

Quite commonly used, these amazing wristbands do the job for many women, but don't get discouraged if they do not do the trick for you. There are so many more ways to help you.

11 Rest, Guilt-free

Afternoon naps have helped me so much during pregnancy to give myself proper rest and attain full energy once I am up. But resting may too require some pointers. It is best not to sleep after having a meal. We don't need to walk around either during these times after meal but watching a little television or reading a book for half an hour and then sleeping would help digest the entire food intake. Good sleep and rest is one the best ways to ensure that we have a good health during these times. It is believed by many, that sleeping actually helps to burn calories especially during the night when body metabolism rate is charged just like a cellular phone that functions and get charged better when not in use.

12 Stay Stress-free

This is simply easier said than done. A lot of mothers work in the early months of pregnancy and with the rising global financial situation. Everyone needs to continue getting paychecks also for the expenses that will be required for the new life which is on its way. The best way to ensure being stress-free and yet earn, is to work from home. If there is no way that working from home is possible, it is advisable to take a break for a while and work from home by free lancing and other stress-free jobs at home. There are many online jobs that are possible at home that could help.

13 Screen Flickers

The continuous working on the computer causes some working mothers to result in morning sickness. The flicker on the computer screen is harmful enough to cause sensitivity in eyes and digestion for mothers. If working on the computer is unavoidable, we can try changing the screen to a soft color that is not bright and harsh on our eyes.

14 Get Loose With Clothing:

Loose clothing like long loose t-shirts even in the first trimester helps prevent morning sickness. There are various maternity dresses available in the market. In spite of being the correct size it may not be loose for pregnant mothers. It helps to wear and go loose on these days. Incase pregnant mothers may wonder what use would these loose clothes come to use, I remember a friend having made so many baby clothes for their baby out of her maternity t-shirts. I thought it was a great idea in various ways.

15 Think Wonderful

I always thought that it was easier to say this and way more difficult to implement it. Reading a book with a soft music in the background does not always appeal to all pregnant mothers. Also, watching romantic comedies and chic flicks may divert minds and prevent depression but it could be temporary. It nice to join a group for pregnant mothers in your area. It helps to share your thoughts and get feeds and ideas about your experiences. But it may not be possible everywhere. Many pregnant mothers write their thoughts down and read them over. They sometimes find it inspiring and sometimes so ridiculous that they laugh it off.

16 The Laugh Meditation

Laughing releases the mothers of tension and women don't have to do it forcefully. I love enjoying my giggles and laughter. Sometimes I find myself laughing about the silliest of things and in turn I start laughing that I laughed. It's the easiest for children to laugh. A happy mother also helps to give birth to happy child. A lot of mothers can indulge in watching funny movies especially family movies. Laughing in turn helps to keep the heart healthy also enabling internal activity in the body. It's nice to join a laughing club during pregnancy as it helps to keep fit the heart and keep it happy.

17 Acupressure and Relief Bands:

The nervous system in our body is said to enable certain pressure points in our body, which when massaged and applied pressure on has a lot of benefits for pregnant mothers and also to fight morning sickness. It is best to seek expert help and recommendation for this. It is scientifically proven to be effective and requires direct physical contact.

18 Scents

Sniffing a little bit of flavored substances can help. Some mothers smell lemons while some may smell coffee beans. Sometimes smelling your favorite softly flavored lip balm also helps.

Using Nutrition or Detox Against Morning Sickness

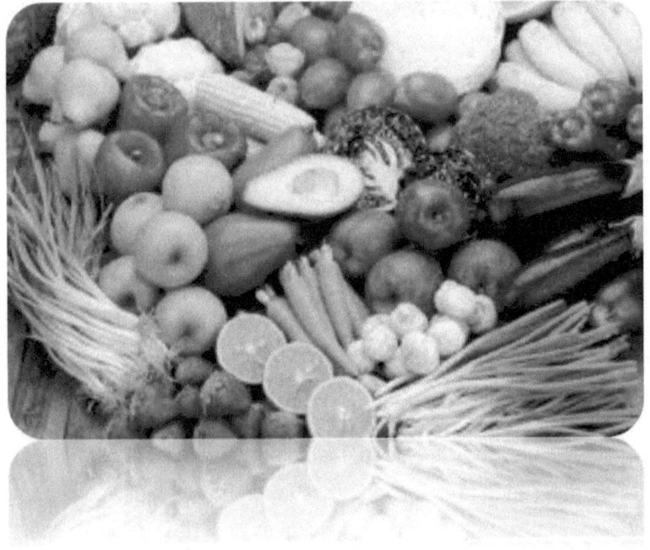

Healing Morning Sickness with Nutrition

High quality nutrition may be the best approach to combat morning sickness because it can work at different levels at the same time. We could summarise the causes into three categories. There may be:

* Specific nutrients lacking in your diet, i.e. too little of something specific.
* Toxicity in your body, i.e. too much of something
* Insufficient calories, simply stated you're not eating enough. The latter can become a vicious cycle: because you feel nauseous, you don't eat, and then again become more nauseous from the lack of food in your body.

I'll discuss some aspects of nutrition here and will talk about toxicity in the "Detox" chapter.

Lacking Certain Nutrients

The following nutrients appear to be crucial in morning sickness:

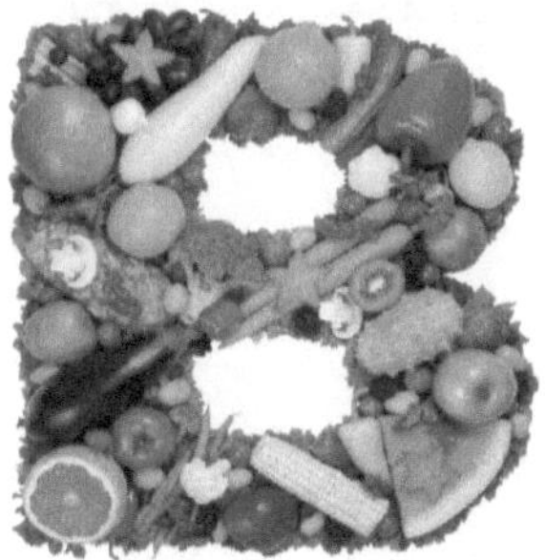

1 Vitamin B6 (Pyridoxine) and Vitamin B12

The deficiency of Vitamin B6 is said to cause symptoms such as morning sickness and vomiting. A healthy and balanced diet may help women recover. Instead of taking Vitamin B6 supplements, women who reported using raw foods with this nutrient have said it helped prevent morning sickness. Some foods with Vitamin B6 that you may try in your diet are avocado, ginger, cranberry juice, citrus fruits such as oranges, vegetables and spices such as clove and aniseed. Vitamin B12 is in fact created in the gut but is also present in dirt. So you ingest it when you eat straight from your garden with some sand attached to your hands, like people did in ancient times. This is risky however if cats use your garden. Wheatgrass, Yeast and Maca Root also are said to help with B12.

2 *Iron*

Iron is one of those minerals that are extra
necessary for our body and a definite one
for us mothers. The reason for that is that
your body has to create a whole blood
system for your baby's body. Since every
haemoglobin molecule contains Iron, a lot
of extra Iron is necessary during
pregnancy. It helps haemoglobin transfer

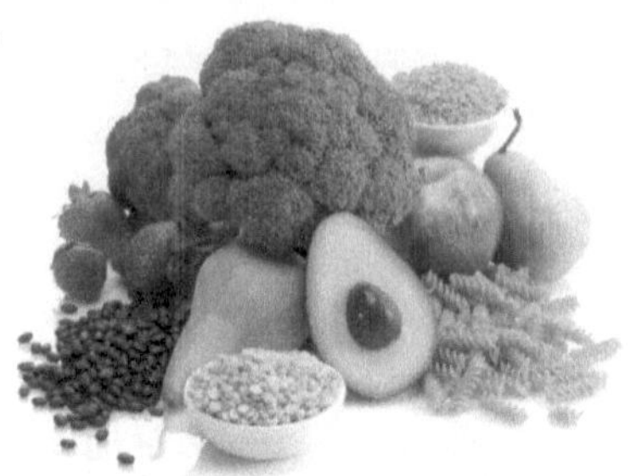

oxygen from the lungs to the blood. One is called anaemic with the lack of
haemoglobin. Since Iron can also be linked to blood pressure which may vary in
the body during pregnancy. Iron is said also be good for the development of the
baby's muscles and strengthen them. Iron simply cannot be ignored in your
pregnancy diet.

3 *Calcium*

Again lack of calcium as a nutrient may not
cause nausea directly for pregnant mothers in
the first trimester but a mother needs bone
strength to sustain the growing baby. I enjoyed
including calcium-rich vegetables in Green
smoothies to make sure I get enough calcium.

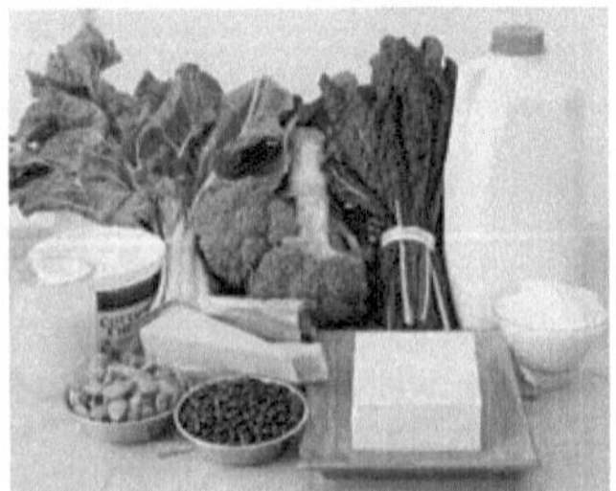

4 *Magnesium*

Magnesium helps absorb the most important nutrients which are Vitamin B6 and B12. Wheatgrass is perfect as a source of magnesium and other raw foods that include it are green vegetables, aniseed, cranberry juice and of course Maca Root.

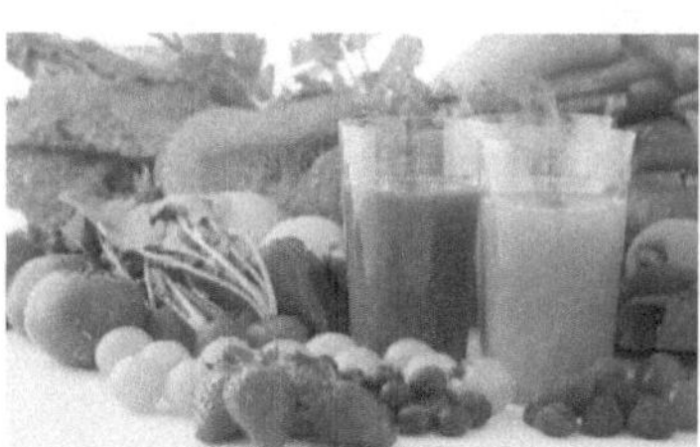

Insufficient Calories

Calories play a part in normal nausea. When a person does not eat enough, they sometimes start to feel nauseous, for example when dieting. This is why having some cookies there at your bedside to eat right after you wake up helps. The body has not taken anything in during the night so your specific morning nausea may just be an expression of your hunger.

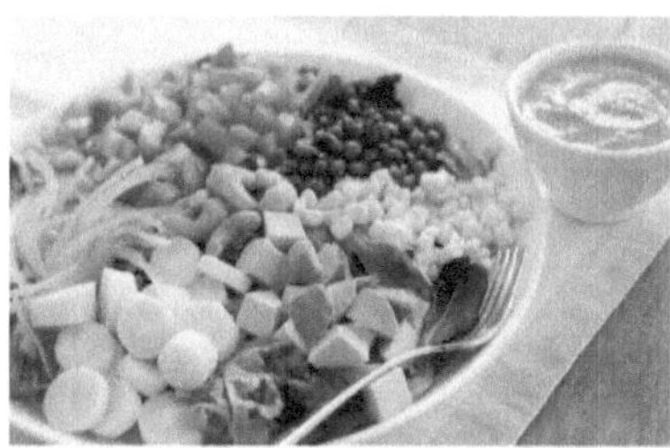

Calories can be taken into the body in the form of proteins, fats and carbohydrates. Next to providing the body with energy, carbohydrates, fats and proteins are building blocks of your baby's new body and are therefore a vital nutrient required during pregnancy. Carbohydrates and fats are mainly the fuel, the energy that the body needs to stay warm and perform all its functions.

Including foods that are rich in one or more of these may just be the solution for your particular pregnancy nausea. Nuts and seeds in general contain high protein and fat. Great sources are Chia seeds.
Carbohydrates can be quickly restored with fruit juices. Grains are also generally a good source of carbohydrates, for example Quinoa which also happens to have the highest protein content of all the grains.

Too many Calories
You don't have to be pregnant to be able to know that eating too much can make you feel nauseous. When pregnant, this effect can be intensified because your stomach is smaller because the growing baby exerts pressure onto it. You may be unconsciously eating meals that are too large, or grazing too much throughout your day. Find out quickly if this caused your nausea by trying half-sized meals for a day or two.

The What, Why and How of Raw Food
Raw foods are foods that are uncooked, not processed and not heated over 116 degrees Fahrenheit. They are also called "living foods". When you heat living foods like vegetables and fruits, the enzymes stop to stay functional over a certain temperature.
Enzymes are large molecules that have a certain flexibility which they need to function. Once they are heated over a critical temperature, they form chemical bonds within themselves and because of that, lose their flexibility and therefore their functionality.
Raw foods are able to retain the nutritional value more effectively than cooked or even processed foods because the food is in its natural form and easier for the body to recognise and digest.
Easier said, Raw food is still full of vitality and that is easy to feel after you drink a glass of freshly prepared smoothie or juice

Raw foods generally consist of just vegan ingredients like fruits and vegetables, nuts and seeds.

A Quick Overview of How Raw Foods Are Prepared

Do nothing

The whole advantage of raw food is that you can eat them as they are. Fruit usually comes pre-packaged in its own skin. Peel and eat! Vegetables like celery, red pepper, turnip, and many many more; you can take a bite immediately after you washed them.

Juicing

A fresh juice, made with a juicer, is one of the best way to consume raw foods. With a juice you can take in much more nutrition from fruits and vegetables than you could do by chewing.

Sprouting

Then there are some raw foods that need further processing, such as sprouting for beans or over-night soaking for grains, seeds and sometimes nuts.

Blending

A blender helps you to prepare tasty dishes such as pies but really also helps you to pre-chew your food so it's easier to eat.

Dehydrating

A dehydrator is similar to an oven and with it you can make crackers, breads and cakes, or dehydrate fruits. They are prepared under the critical temperature; hence they tend to retain their functioning enzymes.

Spiralising

If you like eating pasta, there is an alternative for that too. Zucchini can be sliced into pasta-like strands without cooking, with the help of a spiral slicer or also known as saladacco, which can be purchased online. It turns out that wheat-based cooked pasta hardly has any flavour and zucchini based pasta can be quite convincing to pass for the original thing.

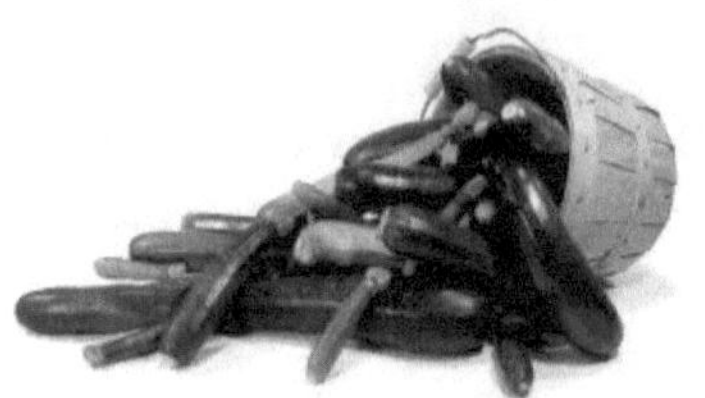
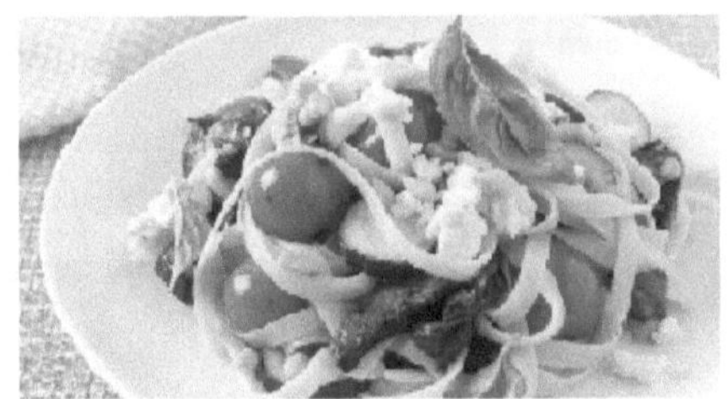

Why Are Raw Foods Important and Beneficial During Pregnancy?

There are numerous reasons why I think raw food consumption helps pregnant mothers battle nausea during those very sensitive days. Here I have listed the most essential benefits of raw foods that I have discovered not only through my own pregnancy experience but through my research over the years. The best part is that most of these raw foods are amazingly delicious!

Uncooked or raw foods help to retain not just digestive enzymes but vitamins, proteins and natural and sufficient percentages of fats. With the intake of raw foods, the need to keep eating more (which can be more psychological than physical) also diminishes and then you have more energy after consuming smaller meals and never feeling uneasy after a meal that makes you feel over-full or stuffed. Raw food has the perfect blend of water, nutrients and fibres to ensure that you get the right nutrition without eating too much.

Raw foods do not require any other agents for taste so the natural flavours of fruits and vegetables are experienced without spices and condiments that could cause a giddy feeling.

Fruits are naturally delicious and some vegetables like cucumber, tomatoes and carrots are not just edible raw but make great salads. Salads are easy to prepare and if a mommy does not feel like chopping them up she can simple wash them and eat them with all the nutritional values intact.

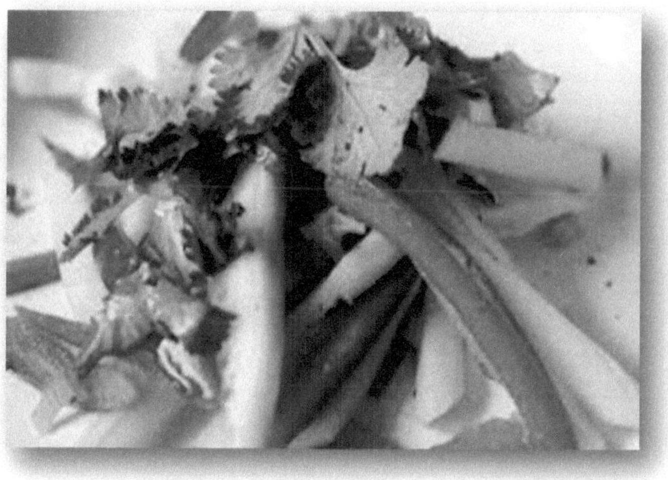

As I mentioned before that raw foods ensure that the food retains its digestive enzymes, it is important to understand how that helps a pregnant woman. The live enzymes present in raw food actually help to digest the food itself. With better digestion, you are ensured that you do not feel giddy or uneasy after meals or even have a reaction of last night's supper with proper digestion and a good night's sleep.

Raw food helps clear bowel movements keeping the digestive system and the metabolic rate up and running. It also helps avoid constipation, a common problem during pregnancy. Better bowel movements and elimination ensures detoxification of the mother's digestive system, making her skin glow and look fresh, besides purifying the blood. But more importantly the toxins in the body that might have caused the pregnancy nausea can be gently removed, and in that way take away the morning sickness.

During pregnancy, women are often less active than usual. This sometimes causes a vicious cycle of anxiety and depression, and too much weight gain due to eating fast food to fight these negative feelings. The extra weight will add another reason for worry.

So, instead of a flavoured soda, mommies can drink fresh juices or simply have a carrot to chew on. Dehydrated fruit slices are a great alternative to munching on oily French fries or chips. They are distinctly palatable and don't make you feel giddy or tired. The added benefit is that these foods do not cause the weight to increase more that what can be expected during pregnancy.

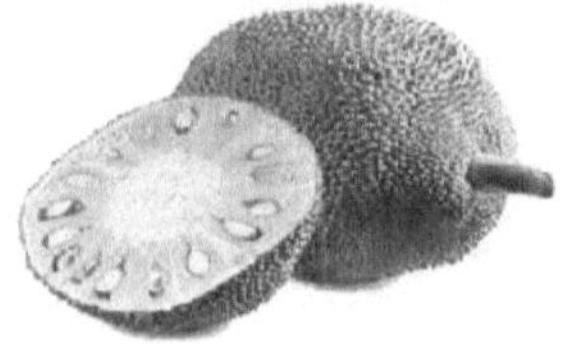 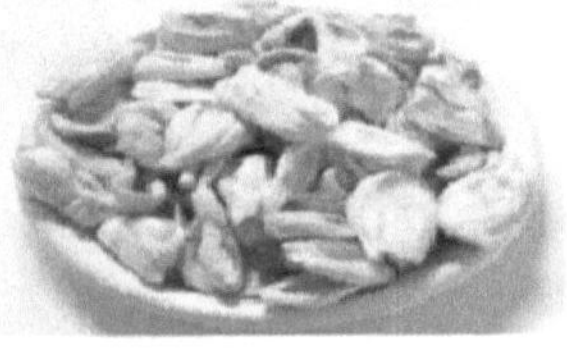

When the body feels energetic and healthy, anxiety causing agents tend to automatically get eliminated. This helps reduce stress for both the mother and the child. If the mother is happy, the baby will feel her happiness and be happier too.

Raw vegan foods like fruits and vegetables have pleasant smell. This is a good thing for pregnant women when the feeling of nausea is mainly caused by unfriendly smells, such as spices and oil in food. The strong smell of some meats, fish and seafood can also cause uneasiness to the sensitive nose of a pregnant woman and lead to nausea and vomiting.

As for salt and sugar, very little or none at all is usually added to raw vegan food. This ensures that blood pressure and the occurrence of diabetes are kept under control.

A word of caution here, because I have heard from many women who have a Raw Pregnancy reacted strongly to the sugar test which uses refined sugar. Raw Pregnant women tend to have increased sensitivity to refined sugar and will show up as diabetic when they take refined sugar for the blood sugar thest. When tested throughout their days, they are not diabetic however, their bodies just aren't used to these large quantities of refined sugar.

If you crave sweets, you could eat dates, fruits or enjoy smoothies and shakes with no added sugar but a more natural sweetener like agave syrup, honey or Stevia. Fruits like kiwi and oranges are fresh and make scrumptious and filling juices that help you stay fit and improve digestion.

Green vegetables are higher in protein and nutrients than fruits and roots and could prevent a pregnancy nausea that might be caused by lack of certain nutrients. I have heard from a women who cured her morning sickness by chewing on celery.

Drinking juices made out of raw green and leafy vegetables like romaine lettuce, spinach and talks like celery, also helps increase the amount of breast milk for mothers. It is important to pick greens that taste OK to you when you eat them just like that. Try various blends of green leafy vegetables along with a fruit to add flavours like apple with a dash of lemon and it makes a palatable health drink, ensuring that once you deliver your baby, you have more than sufficient milk for your infant's growing needs.

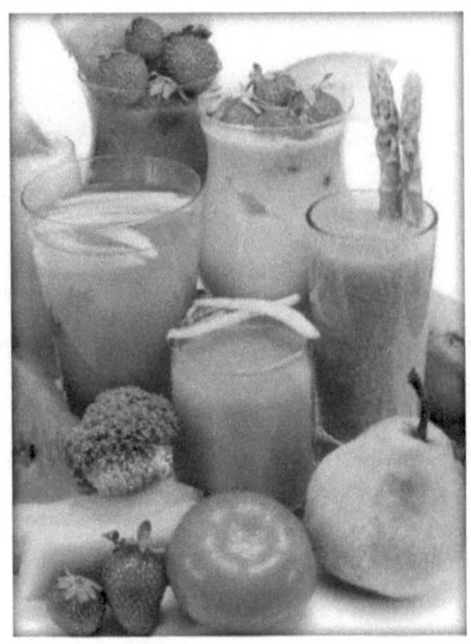

Raw food is pure and unprocessed, apart from being cut or, juiced or blended. The amount or toxins like pestcides that you may ingest with raw food is lower than meat, because in meat the pesticides have accumulated and you get a much higher concentration.

Here's a look at the most beneficial of raw foods and what they have to offer in terms of health benefits:

Food	Vitamins	Minerals	Other Nutrients
Wheatgrass	Vitamin A, E, and B-12	Calcium, selenium, magnesium and iron	Antioxidants, chlorophyll and oxygen content
Maca Root	Vitamin A, B1, B2, B3, C, D and B-12	Calcium, potassium, selenium, iodine, manganese, methanol, copper, zinc, bismuth, magnesium and iron	Polysaccharides, 19 essential amino acids, Campesterol, stigmasterol, beta-sitosterol
Chia Seeds	Vitamin A & C	Calcium, phosphorus, selenium, manganese, copper, magnesium and iron	Omega-3 fatty acids, Omega-6 fatty acids, Protein, Fiber, 8 essential amino acids, Anti-oxidants
Ginger	Vitamin A, B1, B2, B3, C, E, B6, B9	Potassium, manganese, copper, phosphorus, sodium, zinc and magnesium	Gingerols and shogaols, Zingerone, idetary fiber
Avocado	Vitamin B6, E, K	Potassium	Aliphatic acetogenins, monosaturated fats
Citrus Fruits (Common nutrients)	Vitamin C, Riboflavin, Niacin, Folate, Vitamin B6, thiamin	Phosphorus, magnesium, copper, Potassium, calcium	Ascorbic acid, monoterpenes, limonoids (triterpenes), flavanoids, carotenoids and hydroxycinnamic acid, fiber
Cranberry Juice	Vitamin A, C, E, K, Riboflavin, Niacin, Folate, Vitamin B6, thiamin	Calcium, potassium, selenium,, copper, zinc, bismuth, magnesium and iron	Omega-3 fatty acids, Omega-6 fatty acids, Protein, Fiber, Flavanoids
Vegetables (Common nutrients)	Vitamin A	Calcium, magnesium	Folate, fiber
Aniseed	Vitamin A, C, Niacin, Folate, Vitamin B6, thiamin	Calcium, potassium, ,iodine, copper, zinc, magnesium and iron	Protein, Omega-6 fatty acids
Cloves	Vitamin A, K, Riboflavin, Vitamin B6, thiamin, Vitamin C	Calcium, phosphorus, ,iodine, copper, zinc, selenium, manganese, magnesium and iron	Fiber, protein

Cumin	Vitamin A & C, thiamin, Riboflavin, Niacin	Calcium, potassium, copper, zinc, magnesium and iron	Fiber, protein
Fennel	Vitamin A, Vitamin C, thiamin, Riboflavin, Niacin	Calcium, potassium, selenium, manganese, phosphorus, copper, zinc, magnesium and iron	Protein, dietary fiber
Strawberries	Vitamin A, B1,B2, B3,C, E. K and B-12	Calcium, potassium, selenium, manganese, phosphorus, copper, zinc, magnesium and iron	Protein, dietary fiber, Omega-3 fatty acids, Omega-6 fatty acids,

Raw Food V/S Cooked Food

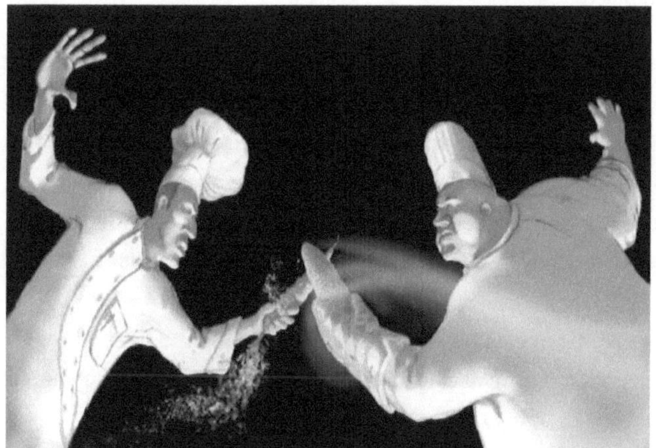

Research has shown that raw food prove to be more beneficial for not just mothers to-be but for anyone, especially the developing foetus. While many people might prefer cooked food over raw options, here's a look at what benefits each has to offer.

Benefits of Raw Food over Cooked Food

The most important factor that is believed to be more beneficial for raw food over cooked food is that the enzymes in food are active when consumed raw but the enzymes are lost and the goodness of enzymes are gone when consuming cooked food. These digestive enzymes help to digest food easily and hence could possibly help to prevent indigestion causing nausea.

It is said, that raw vegetables are extremely low in calories and have an estimated absorption rate of 50 calories in every pound of from raw vegetables.

Despite less movements and exercises during pregnancy raw foods help not to put on excess weight for pregnant mothers. They can rest guilty-free, without worrying about having to lose weight during post-pregnancy and get back in shape.

Cooking is said to destroy close to 50% of the nutrients in any food. When we eat nutritious vegetables or healthy foods cooked, 50% of their benefits are going to waste. So, we may receive very little nutrients despite taking good amount of healthy food and end with incomplete nutrition during pregnancy when consuming cooked food.

Vitamin C is very essential as a nutrient during pregnancy and may be required for making sure that the immune system is strong in spite of the hormonal changes that occur for a mother. However, when cooking foods, Vitamin C is destroyed and hence eating cooked food with Vitamin C does not help. Raw food diets are said to be permit higher retention of Vitamin C and hence improves immunity.

Raw foods taste are natural and hence do not need any hassles with added agents, herbs or spices to prepare. On the other hand, raw foods require spices and even oil, adding to calories and hassles for preparation.

Cooked food requires adding sugar and salt. Salt excess consumption causes Blood Pressure while added sugar may increase blood pressure levels too.

Benefits of Cooked Food over Raw Foods

I came across a very interesting fact about cooked food. We generally add salt and sugar to taste to cooked food when cooking it. When sugar and salt are cooked, they can be less harmful. Cooked Food is simply more palatable.

While raw foods retain natural tastes and flavours, it may not be necessary that they will be delicious and scrumptious to eat all the time. Civilizations have, with time learned to cook on fire. There is a reason for that. It simply tastes better.

Cooked Food at times is easily more digestible for foods that are not edible raw. Vegetables can be boiled and eaten easily. A vegan or raw food diet is not always easy to maintain.

A lot of harmful toxins are prevented from forming when eating steamed or boiled vegetables and healthy food in a soup. The prevention of the occurrence of toxins in the food is said to help absorption, enabling higher nutrient absorption with cooked food at times.

Sometimes cooked food is easier to avail than raw food, we simply can order it over the phone or online for home delivery and don't have to visit the store.

Cooked food can be also bought from stores however with preservatives content which could be unhealthy during pregnancy. It best to eat home cooked food by simply preparing a vegetable soup.

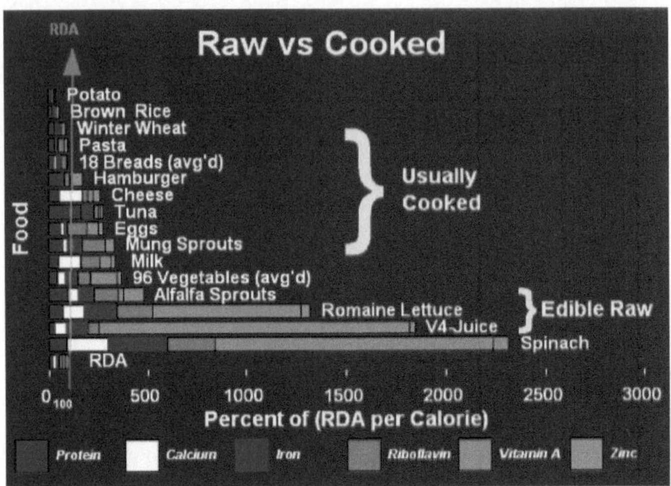

As you can see for yourself, the advantages offered by raw foods outweigh those offered by cooked food. In addition, the smell of cooking or certain types of cooking at least, could have a negative impact on the nausea symptoms.

New Raw Food Cures for Morning Sickness

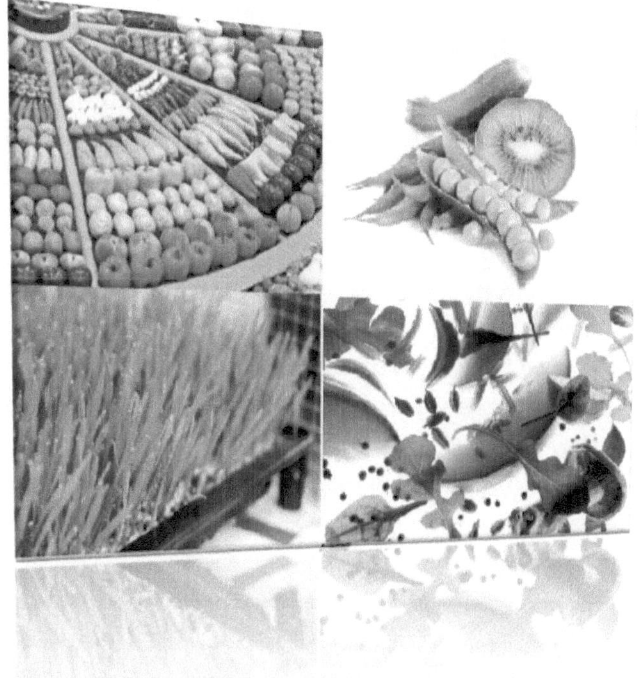

1 The Golden Root

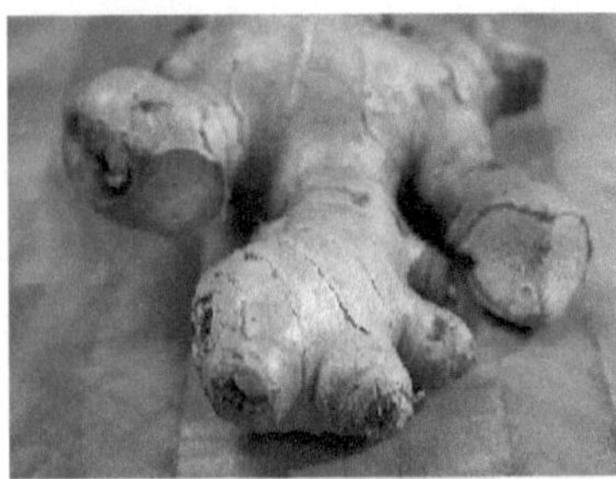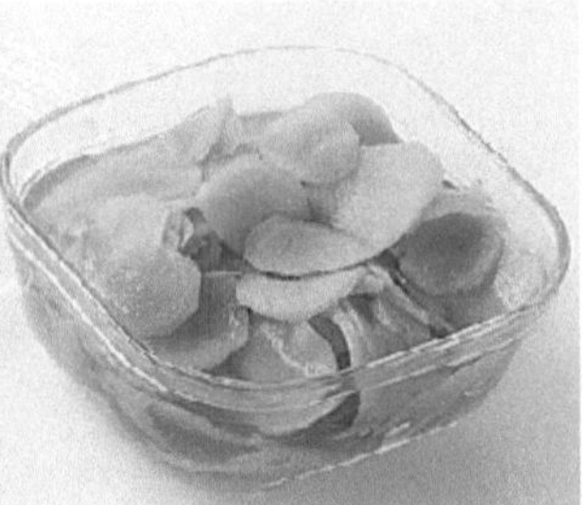

Ginger is an herb that consists of essential chemicals that can help reduce nausea and inflammation and even morning sickness, especially for mothers in their late trimester. According to researchers, the chemicals work chiefly in the stomach and intestines, while also enhancing the brain and nervous system to control attacks of nausea in pregnant women.

The rhizome or the underground stem of the plant is used as a spice along with its medicinal properties. It can be consumed fresh, dried and powdered, or as a juice or oil. I make sure that it is edible first as the taste and the smell is initially very strong and can be a troublesome to consume without soaking in vinegar to dilute some of the strong flavour. Ginger pickle is an option that is great to taste as well as healthy. Despite the fact that it is used as a spice, adding a dash of ginger to lemonade or just making ginger ale could be a great way to have it. It is also great for coughs and colds, and can be added to regular raw food juices for extra flavour.

I have read about ginger having medicinal properties before but was unaware that it is excellent way to fight nausea and morning sickness for pregnant women. I have been adding ginger as a spice to my normal diet ever since I can remember. I'll discuss some additional benefits of ginger here.

- Some studies reveal that ginger decreases nausea and vomiting sensations by 38% before surgeries; hence they are perfect for those pregnant women who by the end of their third trimester are severely prone to nausea attacks.

- It also helps fight fatigue and dizziness. It also a good idea to consume ginger because some women that I have interviewed have said that it helped them recover from motion and sea sickness while travelling during pregnancy.

- Some studies that I came across also show that it helps fight or prevent chronic ailments, such as gout, knee osteoarthritis, rheumatoid arthritis and indomethacin.

- It has properties that help prevent the growth of cancerous tumours and several other fatal diseases.

- Ginger tea is a delicious beverage, which can be prepared by just heating water and adding raw ginger slices with the tea leaves. So, it makes a good ingredient for a raw tea diet as well.

- I also noticed that some studies show that ginger helps in lowering LDL cholesterol due to its ability to decrease the amount of cholesterol absorbed by the blood stream. So, ginger ensures a healthy heart for the mother naturally.

The volatile oils, such as gingerols and shogaols, that ginger contains, are the source of its pungent taste and flavour. The oils help produce digestive enzymes, neutralising the acids that tend to cause nausea, cramps and even diarrhoea in pregnant women.

Use ginger powdered, in a capsule, crushed into a beverage or added to cookies. It's the classical natural remedy and very well known. Didn't work for me though. But you might give it a try.

There is a limitless variety of raw foods available and in general, a diet that contains a lot of raw food may help to relieve morning sickness.

In this chapter however, I have selected a few special Raw Foods that are more effective against morning sickness specifically. I have also listed their benefits so that you can choose the ones that you suspect apply to your specific situation, since the needs of mothers vary greatly from individual to individual.

2 The Magic Root

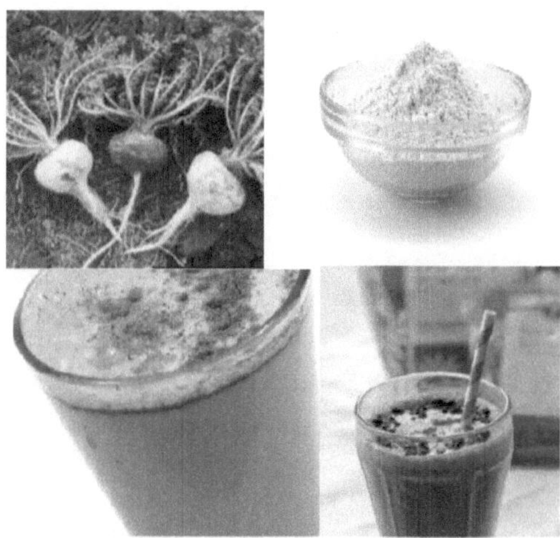

"I began using Maca after I learned that I was pregnant. It is a peruvian root used for thousands of years by Indians in Peru. Since I started using it, my morning sickness is gone & no more bleeding. I understand Maca balances progesterone when too much estrogen is present which causes miscarriages. I was wondering if anyone else has tried is or heard about it? I swear maca got me pregnant."

JazzyLadee08

The other great raw food that is very effective against Morning Sickness is Maca root. The main reason why Maca probably helps is because it helps balance irregularities in the hormones during pregnancy, protecting pregnant woman from uneasiness or nausea caused by drastic hormonal changes.

But it has many additional benefits.

Maca is a root that originates in Peru. It is a tuberous root, resembling turnips, and offers great energizing properties during those exhausting days of pregnancy. Maca is a great alternative for coffee and does not harm the digestive system like coffee does, due to the absence of caffeine in Maca.

Maca Root is grown in the most unfriendly climates on the peaks of mountains. It has been used for hundreds of years, since the time of the ancient civilization of the Incas and the Peruvians consider it a healing food to this day. It was originally used by the people of Peru to boost energy and enhance fertility and libido among men. But it is equally beneficial for women during pregnancy and post-pregnancy.

So, I recommend you to try this natural energy booster yourself. It might give you wonderful results and you may reap all the benefits as part of increasing raw food in your diet. It might not just help you rid yourself of nausea but it keeps your energy levels up during those days when you are normally exhausted by the smallest of exercises like a short stroll in the park.

Maca Root is available in the form of powder to add to make healthy, nutritious drinks. It can be added to other fresh citrus juices like orange juice and even ginger ale, as an energy boosting agent. When you don't like the taste, try adin it to your raw sweet pies. Maca Root can also be consumed fresh like turnips and other root vegetables in salads, chopped or sliced.

It has various other benefits for pregnant women, which we will discuss in the following section but it is important to understand that maca root may very rarely have side-effects.

It may slow down your thyroid, some people are allergic to it, which shows up as hives, fatigue or flushed skin. Other symptoms are menstrual problems, sex drive, upset stomach, heartburn or headaches.

Just start out slow, use organic quality and don't start using other superfoods all at the same time so you know the effect specifically.

I'll discuss some additional benefits of Maca here. The primary note for Maca Root juice has been a wonderful energy booster, beyond anything else. Women who use it do not experience any drowsiness or nausea while consuming Maca during their pregnancy. It may help you overcome giddiness or uneasiness that is otherwise experienced by pregnant women. Here are some of the other benefits I have found through my research:

To start with, for calorie conscious moms, Maca powder servings constitute around 50 calories and there are no elements of fat or cholesterol in its content.

It provides a quick supply of energy for the body, which is very essential for mommies, as discussed earlier.

It also increases the chances of conception and fertility in both men and women. So, just like wheatgrass, consuming Maca juice as part of your regular diet ensures good health for you and your baby.

Maca helps reduce anxiety and stress that often occurs in women when they are pregnant. It can be, as discussed earlier, a very sensitive and stressful period for many women; and Maca actually indirectly acts as an anti-depressant.

Besides energizing pregnant women, it helps improve stamina, which may be later necessary during labour and the delivery of the baby.

It also enhances the immune system by increasing the blood circulation in the whole body, guaranteeing a healthy heart and a strong nervous system, both of which are vital at these times.

Blood circulation also acts as a shield for anaemia, which I found during my research to be a serious and frequent condition among pregnant women.

During pregnancy, women require strong bones to hold the weight of their baby inside their body. Maca helps to improve bone health and strengthen muscles, which in turn help women to bear the child's weight with ease.

Single mothers-to-be face mental challenges, such as managing their lives alone without much help from their partners. However, this is a time when mental health needs to be strengthened. Maca enhances memory as well as mental capabilities of the mother.

Many women have found that their skin glows naturally during and after pregnancy. If you want this glow to persist, incorporate Maca in your regular diet. Maca root improves skin cells and gives a youthful and bright appearance.

Maca Root has a very long shelf life. If refrigerated, its freshness can last up to 6 months. This is why I recommend that to-be-mothers stock up their supply of Maca root powder without worrying about the powder getting spoilt.

Maca Root contains adaptogen properties, which means that it helps the body absorb the right amounts of nutrients, especially for women experiencing hormonal changes.

Maca root with its highly nutritious content and palatability is a great alternative to not just consumption of coffee but it can be added to various other drinks and juices made out of raw foods like fruits and vegetables. Try adding Maca to your raw cookies!

3 The Common Root

The carrot is so common, it can be overlooked in the list of fantastic foods that can , as a glass of carrot juice, instantly cure your morning sickness. It very nourishing, has vitamin K which is great for your baby and could very well be enjoyed daily. Is best taken as a juice, or alternatively grated, as a salad. Great classic recipes are Carrot Apple Juice and carrot Ginger Orange Juice. Drink them every day if you can.

Green Leafy and Stem Vegetables

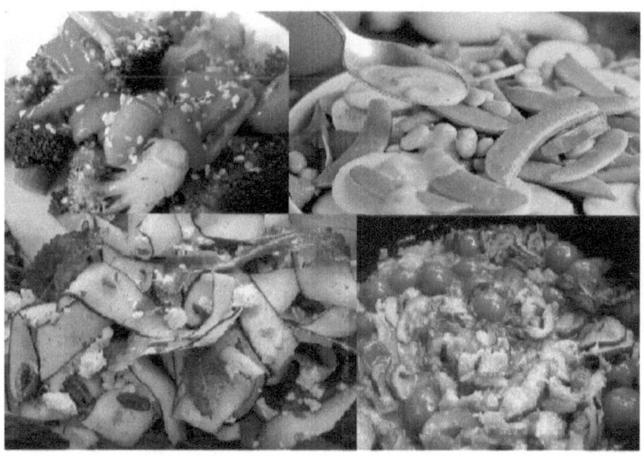

Leafy and stem vegetables are generally more nutritious than the rest of the plant like roots and fruits. Maybe that is why they can be effective against morning sickness. Victoria Boutenko describes these vegetable parts in her book "Green For Life"[1]. They contain more Sodium, Potassium, Vitamin A, B6

---

[1] Boutenko, Victoria. Green for Life. Raw Family Publishing, 2005.

and C. The problem with green leafy vegetables is that most people do not like how they taste. Victoria recommends to blend them with fruits in green smoothies. Its a fantastic way to gets those greens into your diet.

Some other benefits of Greens are that Leafy green vegetables supply fibre and fluid. This helps to avoid constipation problems, ensuring good bowel movements and a healthy digestive system overall.

Some pregnant women experience leg cramps that are best prevented by eating green leafy vegetables. The balanced blend of calcium and magnesium in dark green leafy vegetables is said to fight against such painful leg cramps that can really weaken the mothers during the latter trimesters of pregnancy.

Green leafy vegetables provide an ample amount of iron and folate, which help fight anaemia during pregnancy. A lot of women all over the world are subject to this disease, especially in the developing and under-developed countries, but that does not mean that women in the developed countries need not look after their blood iron levels.

Eating a diet consisting of vegetables could decrease the risk heart attacks, cancer, stroke and even certain kinds of diabetes in pregnant women.

The Vitamin A content in green vegetables keeps your eyesight and skin healthy and may also help to protect against infections.

Veggies barely have any cholesterol content, hence are great for maintaining good cholesterol levels during pregnancy.

There are so many vegetables that can be taken in the form of raw food and are great to eat in the form of salads as well as juices.

1 Celery

" I found a new cure for my morning sickness... Celery... does anyone know why that works?" - Monique on the Raw Pregnancy facebook group.

Celery is one of those common foods that should probably be listed amongst the super foods. Children love it and it helps them to grow. Just give it a try and see if it works for you. Its easy enough to buy a bunch, just wash and cut up in small chunks and snack on them throughout your day.

2 the Power Juice That Instantly Cured my Morning Sickness

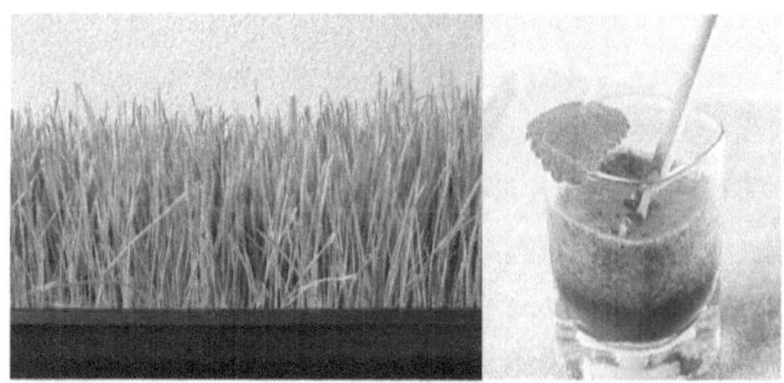

"The wheatgrass came in a small glass and tasted horrific to me. Luckily they served it with a glass of pineapple juice to wash away the taste. The result was astounding: my morning sickness melted away in a matter of one or two hours! And every day that I drank wheatgrass juice, the morning sickness stayed away, the days that I didn't, it came back!"

Patricia de Kuiper

Wheatgrass juice was the one thing I used to help cure my morning sickness and because its effect was so obvious and powerful, it opened up my search for more Raw Foods that might help. And so wheatgrass juice was the inspiration to write this book. As I described earlier in this book, I had a super healthy baby too, and I suspect the amazing nutrition from wheatgrass had something to do with that.

Wheatgrass is grown from wheat berries. The juice has a little hint of sweetness but do not expect it to be as sweet as sugarcane juice. To some people it tastes just fine, to others like myself, the taste is quite bad. Sometimes a dash of lemon helps but I found a great solution to help me with the taste which I'll describe later on.

Why is this juice so powerful? I believe that the main reason why wheatgrass is so powerful against morning sickness is that it is just a very powerful overall quality nutrition. If there are shortages in your diet, Wheatgrass juice will likely take care of them. In general, green juices seem to be very effective against morning sickness which is why I will discuss a couple more later on in this book. In all cases, I believe the core reason why greens are so effective in curing morning sickness is that they take care of basic nutritional deficiencies.

There are so many general benefits of drinking wheatgrass for people in general. You don't need to be pregnant to reap these benefits. But since, we are discussing pregnant mothers and solutions to nausea during pregnancy, we'll focus on its benefits for soon-to-be-mothers here:

Wheatgrass is a natural source of vitamins and antioxidants very essential for the nutrition to newbie moms. It contains vitamins such as Vitamin A, E, and B-12, calcium for the bones, and important minerals such as selenium, magnesium and iron to fight deficiencies often seen in pregnant women that could cause adverse effects for both the child and the mother.

The chlorophyll content in wheat grass juice is as high as 70%. Chlorophyll being a product of light energy from the Sun, through photosynthesis, is the ultimate source of energy for mothers to keep them healthy and fit during pregnancy and post-pregnancy days. Chlorophyll has anti-bacterial properties to keep mothers away from minor ailments like coughs and colds as well.

The brain and all other body tissues experience strengthened immunity with an adequate level of oxygen content. This is what wheatgrass helps with to a great extent.

Several medical practitioners believe that drinking wheatgrass juice enhances the digestive system and is easily digested in the form of a juice. During pregnancy, it helps to enhance digestive immunity of the mother, ensuring the prevention of nausea or sudden giddiness that could lead to vomiting or a feeling of heaviness.

Wheatgrass is said to have amazing medical properties that help restore fertility and enhance the youthfulness of mothers whose bodies are going through drastic hormonal changes during pregnancy.

This green plant naturally protects mothers from blood diseases and increases immunity to ailments that women are prone to due to the hormonal changes during pregnancy.

Wheatgrass juice also stimulates metabolism and the enzyme systems in the body, enriching the blood. It also aids in reducing blood pressure by dilating the blood vessels in the body.

Wheatgrass stimulates the thyroid gland, preventing obesity, which is a serious source of concern for pregnant women, given that they tend to put on weight due to the lack of exercise and the craving for various types of food during pregnancy.

I have a thyroid condition, my thyroid is working too slow. The normal situation during pregnancy is that the body needs more and more thyroid medication as the pregnancy progresses. My doctor was very amazed when he saw that my body needed less and less medication when I drank wheatgrass juice every day.

Overall, wheatgrass leads to increased energy levels, while promoting a good night's sleep, which is great for pregnant mothers who often have sleeping problems. Preventing exhaustion in this way could also be one of the causes why wheatgrass works so fantastically against morning sickness.

If you make your own wheatgrass juice freshly with a special wheatgrass juicer, you can make a paste out of the wheatgrass pulp and apply on your skin and face as a pack. Wheatgrass is said to have anti-bacterial properties as well as oxygen to rejuvenate the skin cells and give a younger looking skin by slowing down the skin aging process.

Wheatgrass also improves eyesight and night vision but that does not mean that we can go gallivanting around the house without switching on the lights at night as a minor accident even at home may cause problems for the child and the mother.

Some tips for growing and juicing your own power juice: You can quite easily grow your own supply of wheatgrass at home and experience its benefits daily without having to run to the market for fresh wheatgrass. You will have to invest in a juicer though, and not just any juicer because wheatgrass is tough and needs something extra to get the juice out. New juicers appear on the market quite regularly. A few suitable brands are Champion, Lexen, any twin-gear juicer and the vertical Hurom type juicer.

All you will have to do is buy a supply of wheat berries (seeds) and get a handful of plastic trays with some soil in which you can grow wheat grass over a week. The wheat berries first need to be soaked for 24 hours, then sprouted for another 24 hours in a sprouting jar. For that purpose, take any glass jar and put the soaked berries inside. Take a small piece of cloth which you attach over the opeining with a rubber band. Rinse the berries twice a day by pouring water through the cloth, then put the pot upside down so that the water can come out. On the third day, spread the sprouted seeds over the soil and make sure the soil stays damp. You can spray or close the tray with a lid, in which case you have to watch out for mold.

Each day, start a fresh batch so you can start harvesting every day after about eight to ten days. Use about a cup of berries every time for one person. By the 8th day, the first cup would be ready to harvest. Cut the grass off as low as possible, there are valuable substances right above the root. This process is not tedious and takes only a few minutes every day and soon becomes a routine.

The best thing is to drink the juice in the morning immediately after making it in the juicer. The juice will start to degrade in about 15 minutes after which it still will be a very powerful drink but why waste a good thing? Drink it as fresh as possible.

Other ways to reap the benefits of this power plant: Even though growing Wheatgrass yourself is a joy to some, to others it seems to be just a big hassle. Me too, I personally enjoy growing it some periods and then feel like it's too much work the next. If you feel like that too, don't let it stop you from reaping the benefits of wheatgrass juice. There are numerous alternative ways, and even though off course standing next to your juicer and drinking it fresh is the very best, don't be a perfectionist when it comes to taking in wheatgrass juice if perfectionism means you will not get any wheatgrass at all, like I have done. Just lower your standard a bit and there's a world of options.

I have sometimes ordered freshly grown wheatgrass and had it delivered in an envelope, by mail, to my home, weekly. Search online if this is possible in your country. The wheatgrass is only one day old when you get it and will stay fresh enough for a week in your fridge. It is a fabulous solution: the wheatgrass juice remains freshly packed in its cells and is in next to perfect condition once you juice it, as long as it is within a week and you keep the grass in the fridge.

The next solution is to order frozen wheatgrass juice online. Just store it in your freezer and add a couple of wheatgrass icecubes to your smoothies.

Another option is dried wheatgrass juice powder. Just add a scoop of raw wheatgrass powder to your smoothies and see if that works for you! Make sure you try this for at least three days to see if it works for you before you move on to try a different solution.

Help! I just CANNOT stand the taste!

If you are bent on taking in the highest quality and want to drink your juice as fresh as possible, it is a real problem if you cannot stand the taste!

It is your luck that I felt exactly as you did, and by accident I stumbled on a great solution to this problem: grapefruit juice. Grapefruit juice magically disguises the taste of wheatgrass! And by the way it does that for other green stuff too for example a superfood like bluegreen algae and any green vegetables in general.

The easiest way to use this is to start by juicing the wheatgrass and then finish by juicing one or two grapefruits. The resulting juice will have every last drop of juice from that wheatgrass in it since you "rinsed" the machine with grapefruit juice. Try it and see if you can stand the taste like this? Otherwise try adding some sweetener like honey or simply try diluting it with water. It really works!

Seeds, Fruits and Berries

1 The Super Seeds That Cure Nausea

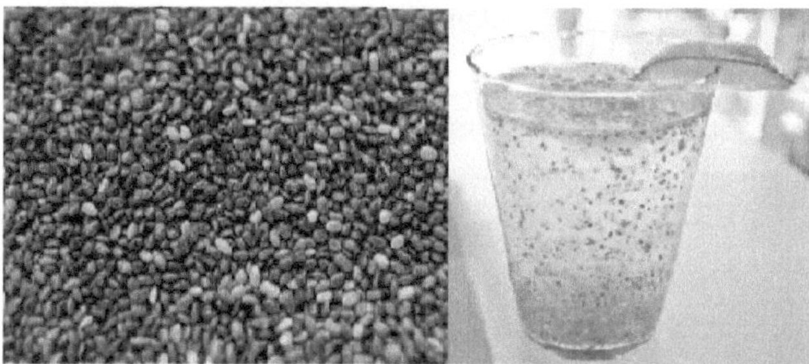

"I guess the Chia seeds fill up my stomach and keep me satisfied, so I don't get that hungry/nausea feeling like I normally do. I can't believe it took me nine months to figure this out! Haha!"

Carrotsnake

The chia seed regime is also an interesting raw food that helps against Morning sickness. It is famous for its high Omega-3 content. The main reason why it works is probably its tendency to take away the feeling of hunger. Chia seeds are mostly found in Southern areas of North America and Guatemala.

Chia is a flowering plant, and can be grown as a house plant. The main reason these plants are cultivated is their seeds. This particular plant belongs to the mint family.

Chia has good nutritional value and a little intake of this particular seeds can fill up the stomach and not make you crave for more food for a long time.

Chia seeds can be consumed as a raw food because they become very easily digestible by soaking them in water for 10 to 15 minutes. Also, chia seeds can be prepared into a gel, in combination with other raw foods. It can also be eaten as a delicious cream cheese made out of other raw foods like avocado and dulse seaweed.

Next to flax seed they are very practical when making raw crackers. Their shell binds liquid therefore helping a raw cracker mix to dehydrate quicker. I like the taste of chia crackers more than flax seed crackers. For any raw cracker recipe that uses flaxvseed, just replace the flax seed with chia seed and you'll have wonderful crackers to munch on throughout the day.

Chia seeds offer a variety of benefits for pregnant women, besides aiding both men and women to lose weight and revitalise the body. Here are some of the interesting benefits that could help pregnant women:
Chia seeds help to lose weight without starvation, since it fills the stomach without introducing a high calorie content and fat. This helps mothers keep their weight in check during pregnancy. Adding too much weight or fat to the body during pregnancy is neither good for the child nor for the mother.

It is important to also maintain blood sugar levels during pregnancy. Several women tend to experience a rise and fall of blood sugar levels during this time. By consuming chia seeds, one can reduce the risk of future development of diabetes.

Chia seeds are a great source of fibre that ensures good digestion and healthy bowel movements, preventing constipation and other digestive ailments that women are prone to during this time.

Omega 3 fatty acids are essential good fat nutrients, mostly available in fish. However, for vegetarians and people who choose a raw food diet, fish might not be an option. Chia seeds are a great alternative in such cases.

These seeds don't need grinding for consumption, unlike flax seeds, and can be easily consumed by mothers without much effort being put into preparation.

It is a good source for hydrating the body for women living in tropical and warm climates, where dehydration can become a serious issue, causing trouble for people in general, not just pregnant women.

It is a great source of protein, which constitutes 20% of its nutritional value. It is also a good source of the 8 essential amino acids.

Chia contains 500% more calcium than milk, ensuring that would-be-mommies have healthy bones.

It also has more Vitamin C than an orange and helps safeguard against coughs and colds.

Iron deficiency during pregnancy can cause anaemia. Chia seeds have 300% more iron content than spinach.

These seeds can also be added to raw food salads and uncooked soups or delicious smoothies very conveniently to be consumed in various palatable ways.

While chia seeds are easily available in the market and can be even ordered online, their nutritional value and goodness have made chia seeds a hot favourite among Western weight loss regimes.

2 The Fatty Fruit

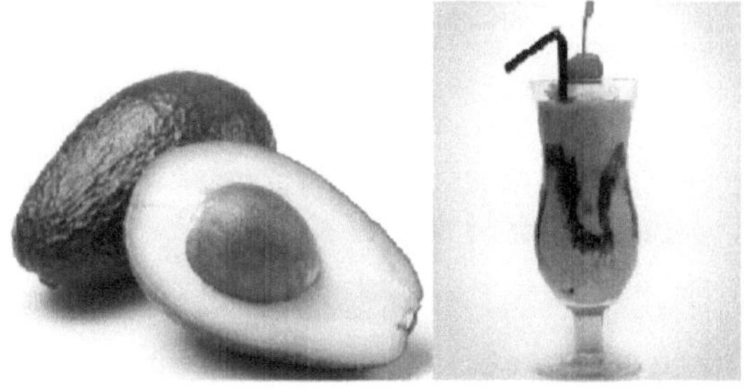

Avocado is a multilevel aid to help you overcome morning sickness: it contains lots of calories from high quality fats, vitamin B6, high in folic acid and vitamin C. There are no known properties of avocado that may hamper a pregnant mother's health and is used by mothers all over the World to overcome nausea and morning sickness during pregnancy.

I have read about it in my studies and realized that the goodness of avocadoes is not just restricted to nausea but other nutritional benefits for a pregnant mother too. Note that avocados need to be ripe, for good digestion hence one can ensure fast ripening, by storing the avocados with other fruits.

There are several general health benefits that I came across in my research for avocado but here are the reasons why I think it benefits mothers who are pregnant and helps beyond a great aid for morning sickness and nausea attacks.

Vitamin B6, present in avocados may be the reasons why avocados help relieve mothers from nausea. I have come across several mothers who have eaten raw avocado to rid themselves for morning sickness.

Adding avocado to a mother's diet is said to also help absorb the nutrients from other raw foods especially vegetables.

The potassium content in an avocado also can help you get rid of leg cramps.

The whole nervous system is taken care of by eating an avocado a day by mothers. It has personally benefitted me too to keep overall nervous system strong and save money on bills for visits to the neurologist during my pregnancy.

Avocados are a great idea, starting from the first trimester as it contains good amounts of folate that is said to be essential for the development of the fetus.

It helps prevent Spina Befida of the foetus: Children with this disorder are born with an underdeveloped spinal cord.

The nutrients from an avocado included in the everyday diet benefits the child and the mother equally when pregnant.

Avocados protect arterial walls against heart diseases and checks the cholesterol levels for a mother. This ensures a mother with a healthy heart too.

Besides all that it does for the health, it is also good for a mother's hair and skin.

Many doctors and mothers have said that they have benefited from avocados in the long run too. Even to reap the benefits for skin and hair, it is best to eat avocados instead of using products with avocado as an ingredient.

3 Citrus Fruits

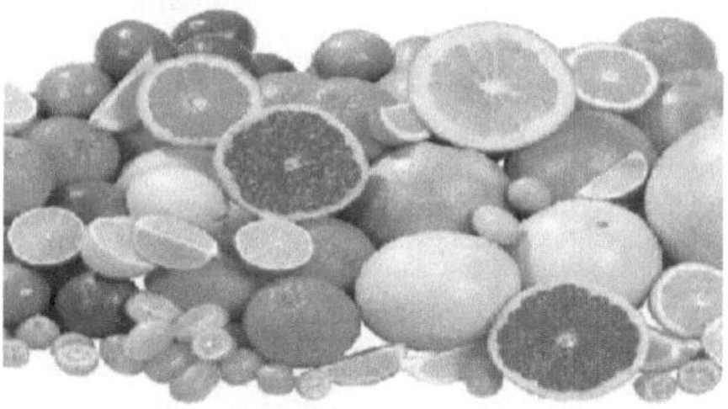 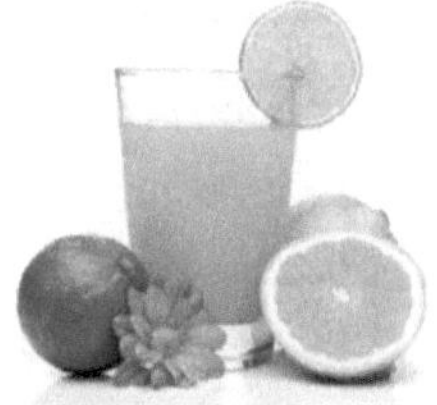

When I was pregnant I thought that raw foods would obviously include fruits because they are the first raw foods that come to one's mind. So, I decided to go all fruity, but citrus fruits were my first choice as a pregnant mother, because I realized that they were not just delicious but also full of benefits that go much beyond Vitamin C and antioxidants to help fight morning sickness.

However, it is advisable to take citrus fruits in combination with other raw foods, since taking them alone might harm the digestive system. Citrus fruits include oranges, lemons, limes and grapefruits, clementines, leech lime, mandarin, kumquats, minneola, tangelo, Satsuma, tangerines and pomelos. They are very refreshing during pregnancy and consist of a compound known as flavonoids, which is said to have anticancer properties. Citrus fruit flavonoids have been found to prevent the growth of cancer cells and the spread of tumours.

I came across an NIH Dietary Supplement Fact Sheet that said that an adequate amount of folate prevents anaemia and birth defects in children. Folate one of the components of Vitamin B and is important for the creation of new cells during the period when the foetus is growing at a fast pace. So, I found out that citrus fruits taken in salads, raw or as delicious juices, along with other vegetable juices, are a great raw food choice that can be taken during pregnancy.

I have already mentioned a few other benefits of citrus fruits earlier, however it is important to understand how good it can be as a raw food for pregnant women.

Enriched with Vitamin C, citrus fruits help ensure a stronger immune system. They are also great for eyesight. As mothers, a stronger immune system is very important to protect the life inside us, which is completely dependent on us.

The vitamin C found in citrus fruits is water-soluble and works as an antioxidant, which protects cells from damaging free radicals.

Citrus fruits also contain Vitamin B6, which is said to keep the nervous system up and running, building new red blood cells for the cleansing of the blood stream and stabilize blood sugar levels, which tend to rise and fall during pregnancy.

As I had mentioned before, flavanoid compounds in citrus fruits help fight the growth of cancer cells. They are also good sources of antioxidants that may be able to protect mothers against heart disease and keep cholesterol levels in check.

Citrus fruits are said to contain water-soluble fibers that help balance cholesterol and blood sugar levels.

Due to the high fiber and low calorie content, pregnant mothers don't gain weight. In fact, it helped me reduce excess weight post-pregnancy, when I included citrus foods with my regular raw food diet.

Please note that citrus fruits are best not taken alone or can be avoided in the morning to prevent gestational diabetes, which sometimes occurs in pregnant women. These are best taken as snacks and juices during the day.

1 Cranberries

The sour cranberries are easiest taken as a juice. It is said to provide mothers with a great immune system, relief from and prevention of urinary tract infections during pregnancy and, most importantly, prevention of damage to the genetic material or DNA during the first trimester of pregnancy.

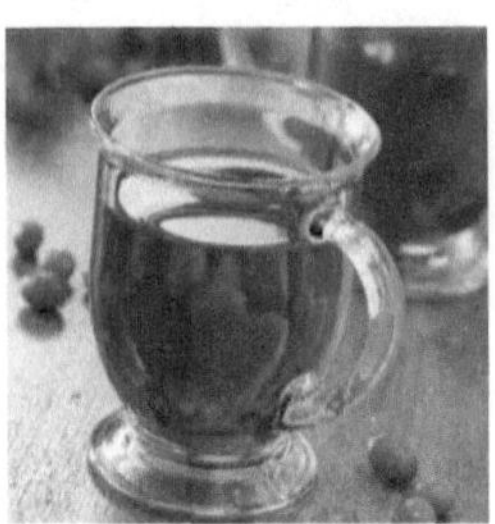

2 Strawberries

Strawberries are perhaps a superfruit when eaten during pregnancy, as it is said to protect children from birth defects. It also helps in the reconstruction of DNA (the genetic map) during pregnancy.

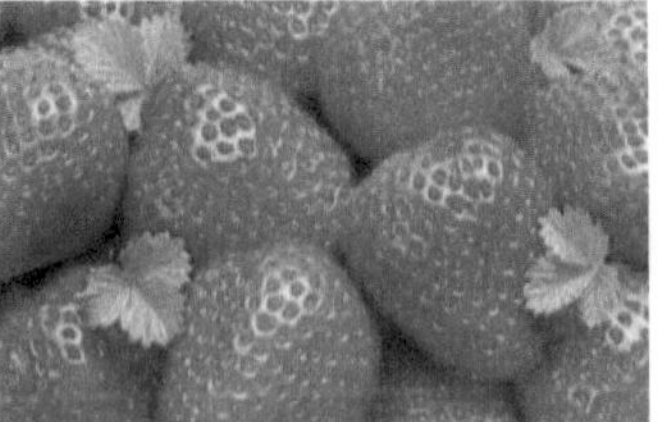

Teas are easy to prepare, and you can make a batch and drink from it all throughout the day, whether hot from a thermos or cold.

1 Ginger

Ginger is the most widely known anti morning sickness remedy. You can make the tea from free ginger slices, dried ginger or even powder. Try seeping it in boiled water but overnight seeping in water in the fridge may work just as well. Don't be discouraged if Ginger tea does not work for you. just try the other remedies listed in this book.

2 The South American power Tea

My friend herbalist Roell Kerkhout advised me to try Abuta, a herb that is used widely in South America for all kinds of women's problems. I tried it and found that its power to cure morning sickness is absolutely amazing.

During my second pregnancy, I had a hard time picking up my wheatgrass –juice routine and found that I didn't mind my morning sickness so much that I wanted to end it. It was just an incidental morning sickness here and there, mostly when my body was uncomfortable from cold or hunger. So I didn't do much about it except to stay warm and fed. But, one night I woke up at 3 am with a strong nausea which seemed to come out of nowhere. It was defenitley too much to handle and I went down into the kitchen to try that Abuta herb which had been standing in my cupboard for a while. I boiled some water and poured it over some loose Abuta herb which I had put in a cup. Then let it seep while waiting until it had cooled enough to drink. The result blew me away: my morning sickness disappeared like melting snow; in a matter of one or two minutes it was just GONE! I couldn't believe how powerful it was!. So I decided then and there that it was definitely going into the morning sickness book.

3 Cumin

Cumin has positive effects on the digestive
system. Try seeping cumin seeds in tea, with
1 teaspoon of cumin and a hint of nutmeg.
This effectively helps to recover from stomach
problems

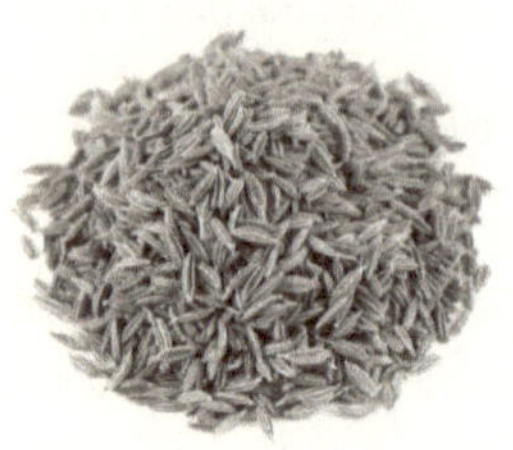

4 Clove

This is another great nausea-fighting tea. Please
remember that the water should be boiled before
adding the spice, so as to only heat the spice and
not cook it. I once tried adding clove flavouring to
orange juice. It was not a bad result at all. Cloves also help to fight sore throats.

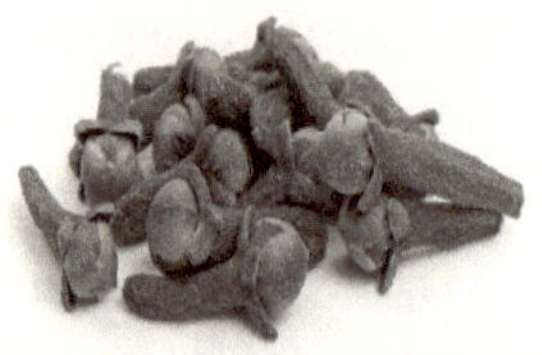

5 Fennel

This is also a great ingredient for tea. It can help
reduce feelings of nausea. You could add a few
drops of honey to make the tea sweeter.

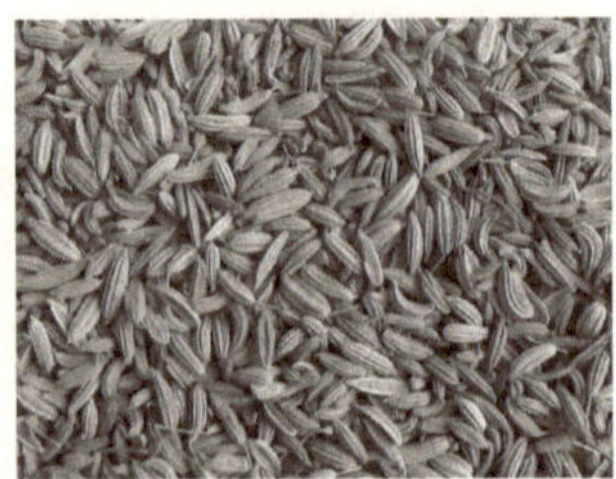

6 **Aniseed**

This beautiful star-shaped spice is said to give instant relief from nausea and vomiting in general.

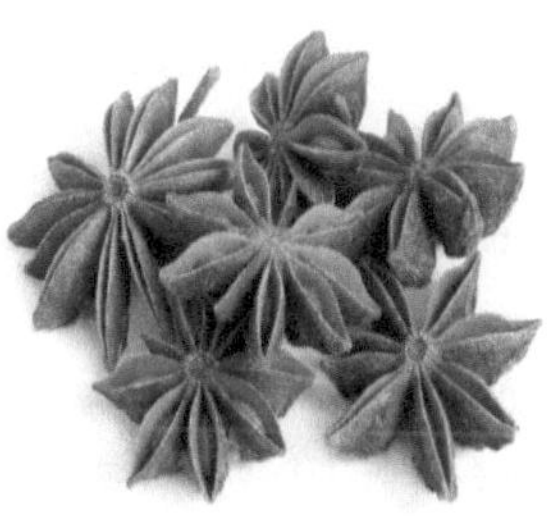

7 Raspberry Leaf

Raspberry helps the pregnancy in general by supporting the uterus. It may help your body just so much as to relieve the nausea.

Toxicity

Since certain types of fasting help against morning sickness, it must mean that toxicity in your body may be the cause of your pregnancy nausea. You need a diet that is clean and helps your clean out your intestines. Raw Food does all of that.

Fibre aids in cleaning the colon. Dietary fibre is made up of cellulose. It acts like little brushes that sweep your digestive tract clean and help your body to get a grip on the other nutrients. In that way it can help to detox the body on a daily basis. When the colon is clean, it helps enhance the overall health of a mother to be. Since an oversensitive digestive tract is thought to be one of the causes of morning sickness, keeping the digestive track clean with a high fibre diet like the Raw Food diet makes much sense.

Fresh Organic Raw Vegan foods in general tend to stimulate the liver to start to detox. Just increasing such foods in your diet may gently detox you enough to get you over your morning sickness.

Detox in general is usually advised against because the toxins that are released in the blood stream are supposed to intoxicate the baby.

However, this is largely a theory and I have yet to see the evidence for it. However mild detox processes that I will discuss later have shown to cure morning sickness, increase energy levels and produce strong babies.

Most women that I've talked to feel weary about doing a detox while pregnant. The fear is that the toxins that were stored in the body tissues, will end up in the bloodstream poisoning the baby. There seem to be two camps: experts and pregnant women who have no experience with detox during prengnancy who advice against it on one side, and women who went raw during their pregnancy or detoxed otherwise, who's baby turned out to be in super health. I have personally gone raw during my first pregnancy and my baby turned out super healthy too.

So, the fear of detox during pregnancy may not be grounded at all.

1 Raw Food in general will detox your body

Just eating a raw organic balanced diet will gently start detoxing your body. Often this diet will make the nausea disappear by itself.

2 Three-Day Method

"One lady mentioned her Doctor telling her to a three day watermelon fast for morning sickness, and apparently it completely worked for her!" – Suzanna in the Raw Pregnancy group.

If a three-day melon fast helps to cure morning sickness, then that means that there was some toxicicy in the body that caused it. I have not heard from other types of fasting exept the melon fast. Better stick to the winning strategy: if a melon fast works for others then why not try it yourself?

3 Oil detox method

Oil pulling is a widely used strategy for clearing up many ailments and diseases. A friend of mine used only this method, to keep her nausea at bay. She had to do it three times a day and if she skipped or was late, the nausea came back and reminded her to oil pull.

Just take one or two teaspoons of either coconut oil or sesame seed oil in your mouth and swish it around for about fifteen minutes in your mouth. Do not swallow it!. After fifteen minutes, spit it out in your organic waste bin to your toilet.

A Diet Plan for You

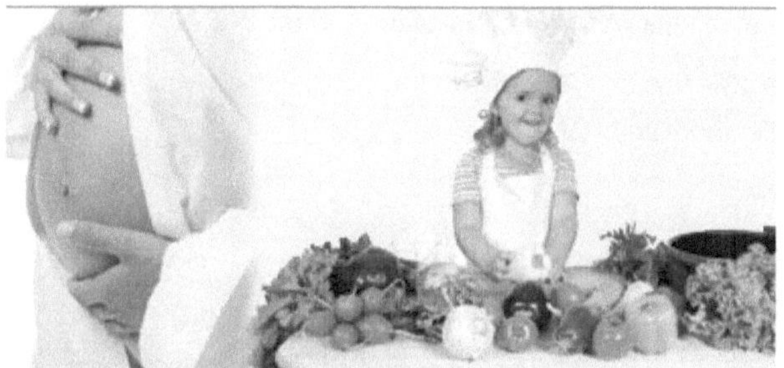

Why You Need A Personal Plan

Food choices are very personal. You have your own preferences for flavour and on top of that some of the remedies described here will work fantastically while others will do absolutely nothing for you.

Sit down for a moment and write down any symptoms you're experiencing. Include all of your symptoms, even if you don't think they're related.

write down those moments when your nausea was worst.

Now, from the life style tips and remedies in this book, write down a list of those remedies you'd like to try first.

Take into account:

- **Nutritional Value**

- **Taste and Flavour**

- **Results**

- **Diet Maintenance Factors**

How To Create A Personal Diet Plan

Here is a step by step process on how to create the diet plan, implement it and finally manage it in accordance to the earlier mentioned factors. It has been quite simple and easy for me to maintain and am sure that you'll fun while working on it.

1. Use a one page per day appointment book available in stationary shops. If you have a exercise book or a planning diary too that too would be easy to fill.

2. Write down all that you eat, the quantity and how it made you feel after eating them.

3. Make a menu plan for a week

4. Replace the recipes that did not taste well or those that did not make you feel great afterwards, with new ones.

5. Then you could write down how you find the new recipes.

This helped me plan, implement and manage my raw food diet plans during pregnancy. It is the least cumbersome way and you could actually be able to research the ingredients by application and experience just like my friends and I did.

Raw Food Recipes

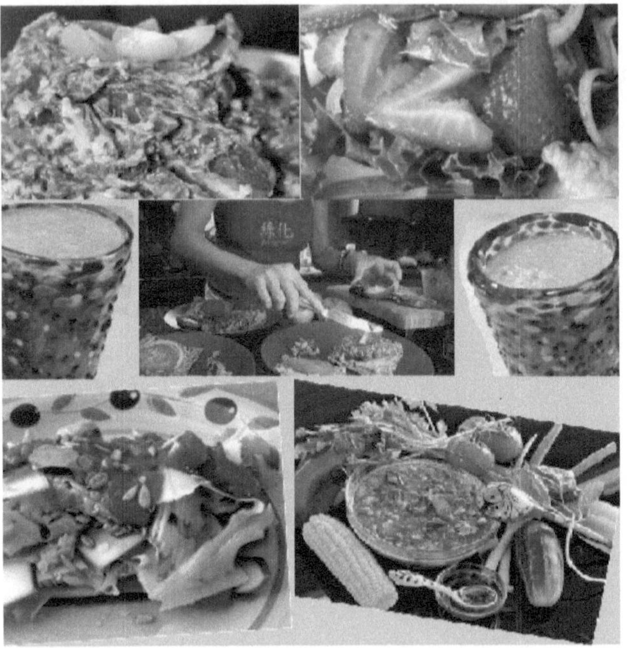

These recipes contain ingredients that were discussed in this book. I have divided them into 5 main sections, each containing 3-6 great recipes:

- **Juices and Smoothies**

- **Breakfast**

- **Lunch/ Dinner**

- **Snacking Time**

- **Desserts**

Green Juice

Ingredients:

- 3 stalks celery

- 2 medium cucumbers

- 5 fresh spinach leaves

- 1 tablespoon mint leaves

- 2 ounces fresh wheatgrass

- water

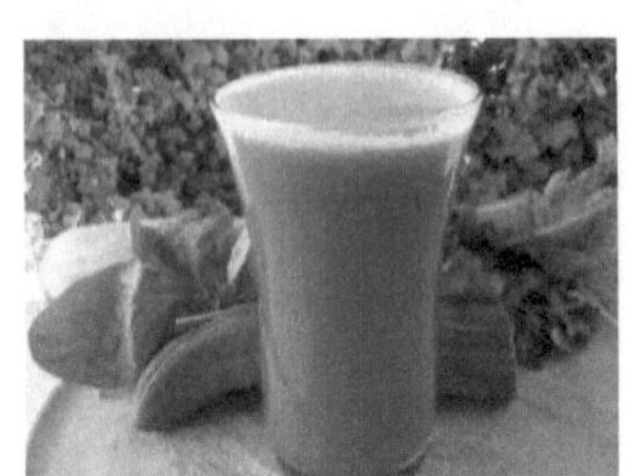

Directions:

1. Chop the celery and the cucumbers into small chunks to fit into the juicer.

2. Start blending in the juicer.

3. Add Spinach leaves.

4. Start blending again, followed by adding mint leaves as per taste.

5. Add Wheatgrass and blend.

6. Dilute with water for texture and taste.

Mixed Fruit Smoothie with Chia Seeds

Ingredients:

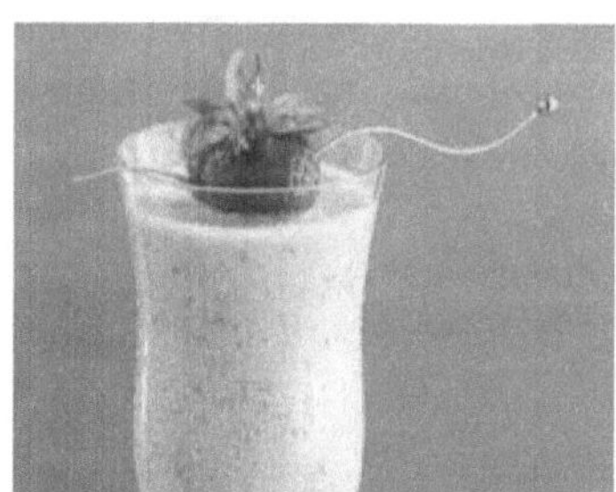

- 1/4 cup of strawberries
- 1/2 cup of blueberries
- 1 peeled and seed removed orange
- 1 ripe banana
- 1/2 cup of fat-free plain yogurt
- 1/2 cup of tofu
- 2 tablespoons of chia seeds
- 1 tablespoons of agave nectar

Directions:

Blend all the ingredients in a blender until it is a thick smoothie. Add water if you find it necessary to dilute.

Maca Blackberry Smoothie

Ingredients:

- 1 cup of coconut milk tonic/ milk/ liquid of choice
- 1 – 1 1/2 cups of frozen blackberries
- 1 banana (ripe)
- 1 tablespoon maca powder

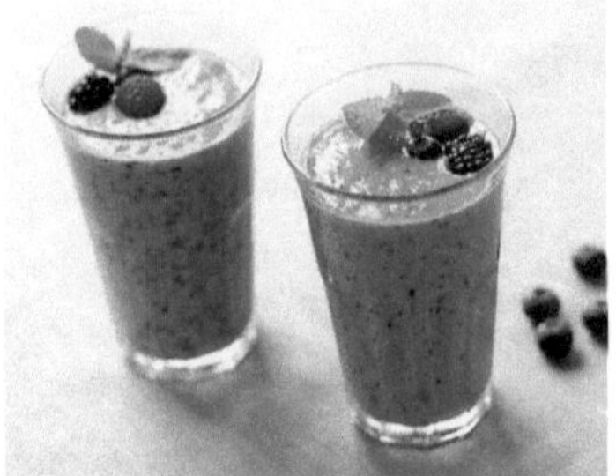

Directions:

Blend the ingredients well in the blender and enjoy this refreshing smoothie at any time of the day. Please note that the portions are sufficient for two people.

Fennel Mocktail

Ingredients:

- 1 fennel
- 2 apples
- 2 handfuls of spinach
- 1 pear
- 1 mango
- 1 celery stalk
- 1/2 chopped piece of ginger

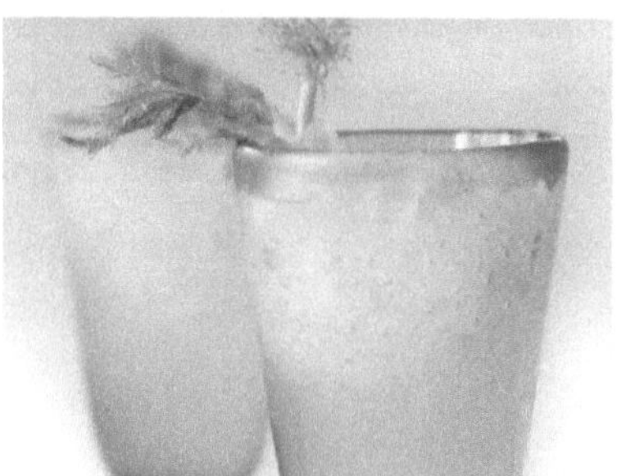

Directions:

Juice all the ingredients to make a delicious drink that is both nutritious and great for pregnant mothers with nausea problems. This has fine anti-nausea ingredients such as ginger and fennel and vegetables that include celery and spinach. The fruits add taste. I personally found this drink very scrumptious to taste.

Carrot Juice

Ingredients:

1 portion of washed and peeled large carrots

1/2 lemon (peeled)

2-3 leaves of lettuce or other leafy greens

1 apple

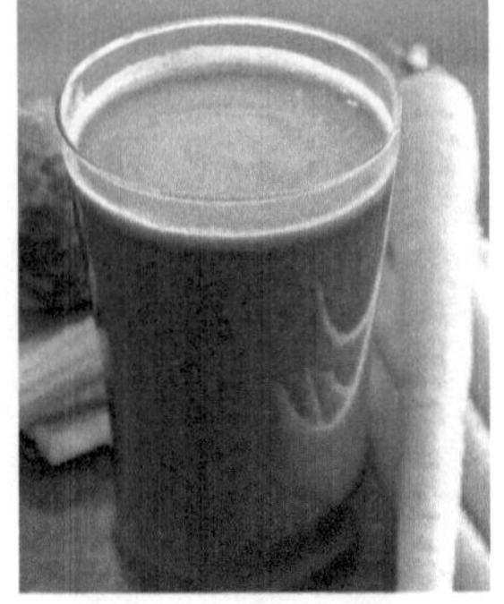

Directions:

Mix all the ingredients into a juicer and preferably use a centrifuge juicer for carrots. This particular recipe is great for pregnant as well as lactating mothers and is said to help enrich the overall health and skin needs of mothers.

Raw Strawberry Banana Crepes

(Will need a Food Processor and a dehydrator)

Crepes:

Ingredients:

- 4 Bananas

- juice from 1 lemon

Directions:

1. Add the 4 bananas into the food processor.

2. Add lemon juice and process the ingredients until it's a liquid.

3. Pour the liquid into 5inched round circles.

4. Spread the mixture to avoid lumps.

5. Dehydrate overnight at 115 degrees and avoid over drying them.

Cashew Vanilla Cream Wraps

Ingredients:

- Coconut pulp from young green coconuts

- 1 cup of soaked overnight Cashews

- Drops of Vanilla Essence

- Store-bought Raw wraps

Directions:

Blend the cashews with the coconut pulp and vanilla essence. Refrigerate if thickening is required.

How to Serve:

1. Spoon the Cream into half the wrap.

2. Add more cream.

3. Fold the crepes.

4. Add ripe berries on top, for garnishing and taste.

Carrot and Lemon Cups

Ingredients:

- 2 cups of finely grated carrots

- 1 tablespoon of lemon juice

- 1 teaspoon grated lemon zest

- 1 teaspoon extra-virgin olive oil

- 4 juiced lemon halves

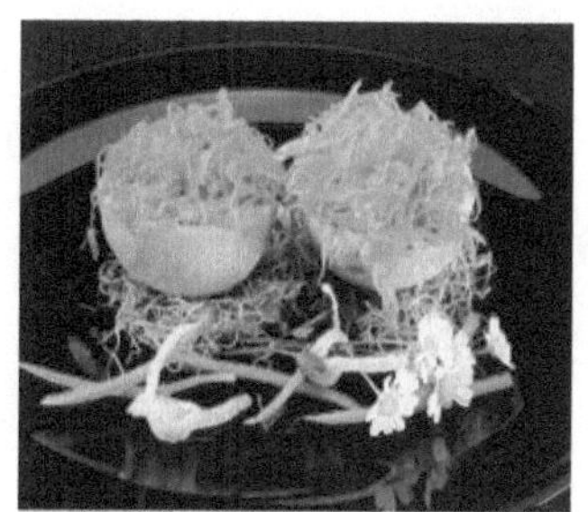

Directions:

1. Grate the carrots.

2. Ina mixing bowl, add all the ingredients

3. Fill the lemon with the carrot mixture

4. Serve with maple syrup for added sweetness

Orange Chia Seed Breakfast Pudding

Ingredients:

- 1/4 cup almonds (must be soaked overnight, drained and rinsed)

- 1 cup water

- 3 dates, softened with pits removed

- 3 oranges

- 1/3 cup chia seeds

- Granola for topping if desired (from Raw Transitions)

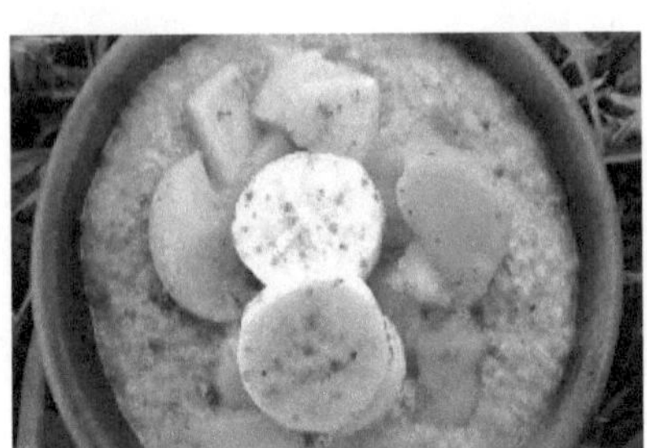

Directions:

Add water with almonds in a high-speed blender until it forms a rich thick paste. Strain the almond milk. Add the almond milk with dates in the blender. Blend into a smooth mixture. Add the orange zest to the almond milk date mixture. Please note to segment the insides of the orange and set aside. Make a juice of the remaining oranges. Add half a cup of the juice to the almond milk mixture. Start stirring the mixture after adding the chia seeds and set the mixture aside for 20 minutes. Add granola toppings for taste.

Lunch/ Dinner

Burrito de Raw

Ingredients:

- 1/2 cup walnuts, soaked and drained overnight
- 1 green onion
- 1/4 cup of sundried tomatoes
- 1/2 an avocado
- 1/4 teaspoon of sea salt
- 1/4 teaspoon of garlic powder
- 1/2 teaspoon of cumin
- A dash of cayenne pepper
- 2 large romaine lettuce leaves for the "tortillas"

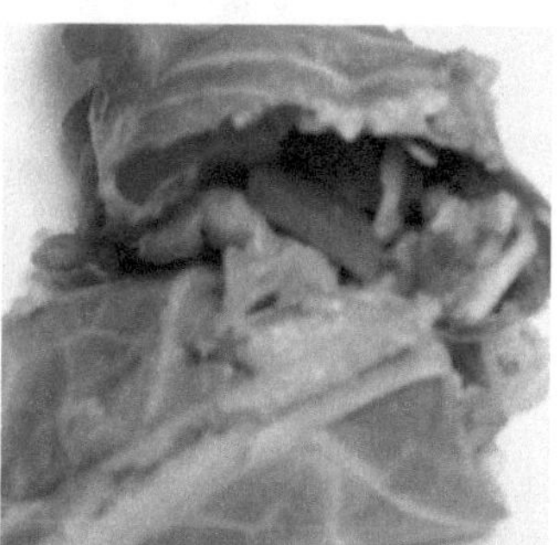

Directions:

We could begin by soaking walnuts in spring water overnight to enhance digestibility. Drain the walnuts. Chop all the ingredients into chunks and mix well together except the lettuce leaves for the tortillas. We need to then spoon the mixture into the center spines of lettuce leaves resembling tortillas. Roll sides up like burritos.

Chipotle Corn Soup

Ingredients:

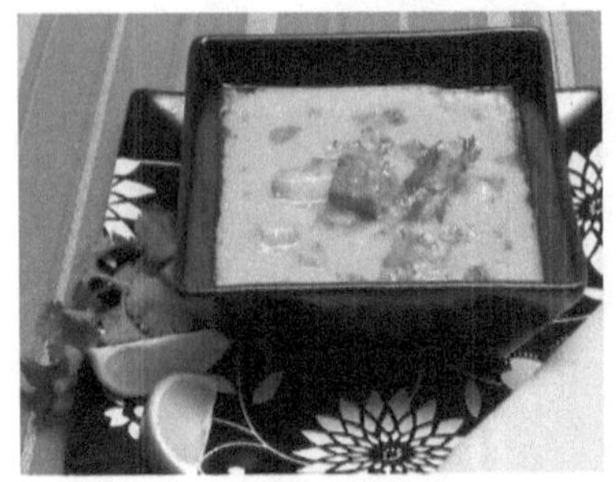

- 4-5 cups fresh corn

- 1 1/2 cups of water

- 1/4 of teaspoon chipotle

- 1 pinch of Himalayan salt

- 1 pinch smoked paprika (optional)

Directions:

Blend all the ingredients except the paprika until combined. Strain the mixture. Serve topped with a pinch of the smoked paprika and kale chips.

Sweet Tomato Basil Soup/ Gravy

Ingredients:

- 1 cup of cherry tomatoes

- 1/2 an avocado

- 1 Tablespoon fresh basil

- 1 small clove garlic

- 1/4 teaspoon sea salt

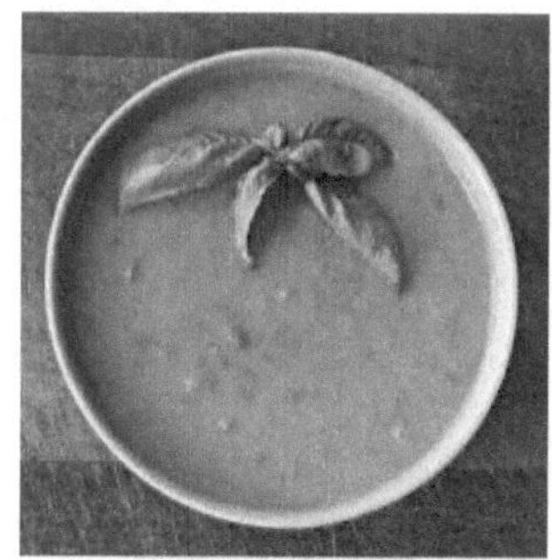

Directions:

Use a blender or a food processor to mix all the ingredients. This is a very good dish and if you want to make gravy out of it, instead of a soup, you can try leaving it a little chunky. You could make some pasta out of the zucchini with a thin strip-slicer and garnish it with the gravy for a different kind of dish.

Kale Low-Cal Salad

Ingredients:

- 4 cups of deveined and finely shredded Kale 1 cup grated carrot
- 1/2 cup of shredded mint leaves
- 1/3 cup of cranberries
- 1/3 cup of sunflower seeds
- 3 Tablespoons of Olive Oil
- 1 crushed clove of garlic
- Sea salt and pepper to taste

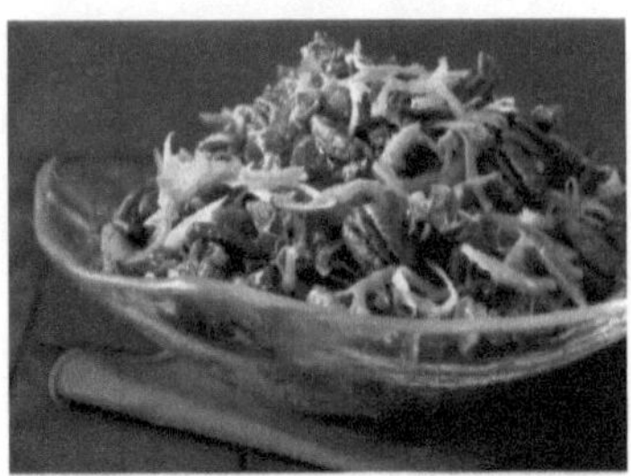

Directions:

Mix up all the ingredients and the salad is ready in no time. This particular salad is great for light meals or lunches. It isn't very heavy and keeps the stomach full. Kale leaves need to be softened before mixing it up with the other ingredients. The best part is that it tastes better, the next day it is prepared. So, you can always eat the left-over for later on, or as a snack.

Tap-a-Tapioca Pudding

Ingredients:

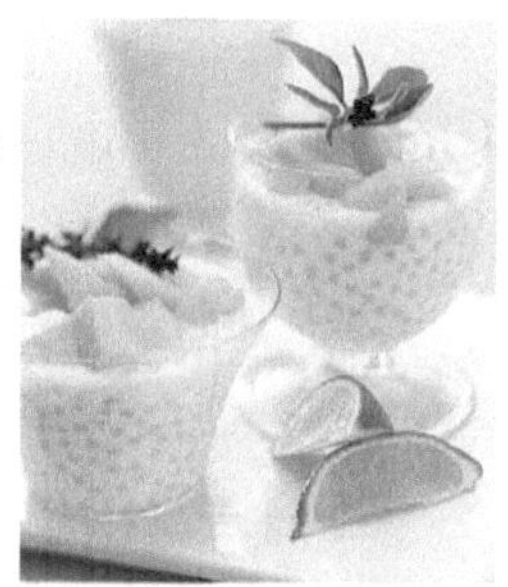

- 1 cup raw nut milk (your choice but I personally like almond milk)

- 2 tablespoons of chia seeds

- 1 tablespoon of maple syrup

Directions:

Mix the raw not milk and the chia seeds together along with the maple syrup. Stir well to avoid lumps. Let the mixture sit for an hour. The chia seeds will bloat up. The scrumptious pudding is ready in no time.

The Veganilicious Burger

Ingredients:

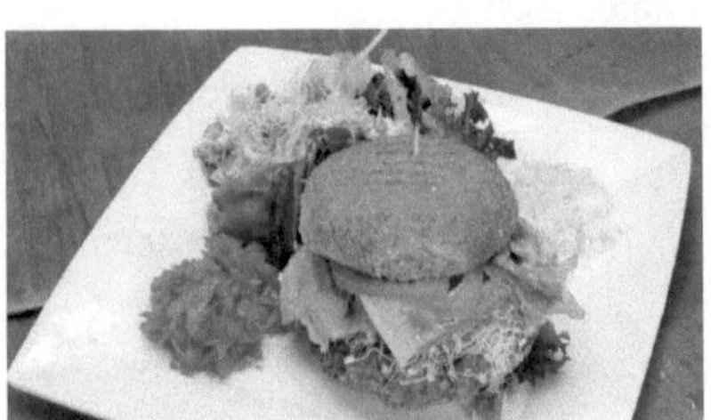

- 2 cups of mushrooms

- 1/4 cup tamari

- 3 carrots

- 1/2 a beetroot

- 1 stalk of Celery

- 1cup of hazelnut flour

- 1/2 cup grounded flaxseed

- Basil to taste

- Thyme to taste

- Few leaves of romaine lettuce

Directions:

1. We would need to peel the beetroot and the carrots before using them.

2. We then need to mix and process all the ingredients in a food processor.

3. After processing the mixture, we need to make round small burgers out of it.

4. We need to then dehydrate the burgers for around 4-6 hours.

5. Spread some raw sour cream

6. We then can cover the burger up in a romaine lettuce.

7. We can also add some avocados or olives as toppings, finally rolling up the burger inside the lettuce and we are ready to go!

Raw Pesto Stuffed Mushrooms

Ingredients:

- 15-25 washed and stemmed button mushrooms,
- 1 cup of slightly chopped walnuts
- ½ cup of chopped pine nuts
- 2 cups of shredded basil leaves
- ½ cup of extra virgin olive oil
- 3 cloves of finely chopped garlic
- ½ t sea salt

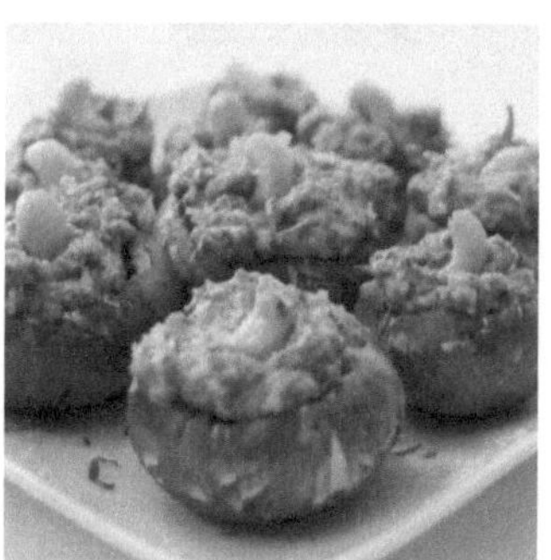

Directions:

1. Place mushroom caps on a dehydrator tray with the top side down.
2. Blend the stuffing ingredients in the food processor.
3. Scoop and fill in a small amount of the stuffing into each mushroom.
4. Dehydrate at 105 degrees for 5-6 hours.
5. I have tried it with a green salad and it's a perfect snack for all expecting mothers!

Collard Green Wraps

Ingredients:

- Collard Greens

- Green onion

- Tomatoes for garnishing

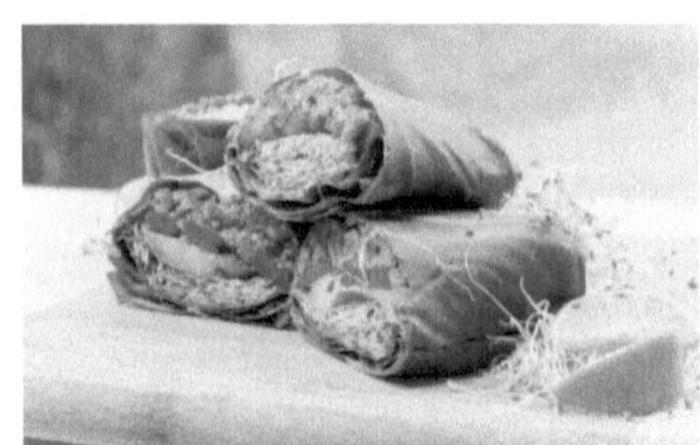

Filling:

- 1/2 cup of soaked hazel nuts

- 1/2 cup of soaked sunflower seeds

- 1/2 cup of soaked almonds

- 1-2 sticks of chopped celery 1/2 cup of water

- 1 tablespoon of virgin olive oil

- 1 tablespoon of agave nectar

- 3 tablespoons of lemon juice

- Salt to taste

Directions:

1. Process all the filling ingredients in a food processor.

2. Spoon and fill 2-3 tablespoons of the filling in each collard green.

3. Tie 1 green onion around the collard wrap to hold the wrap together.

4. Add garnishing of chopped tomatoes.

I personally am very fond of this wrap, which goes great with wheat grass juice as a complete evening snack.

Raw Onion Crackers

Ingredients:

- 2 cups almond pulp leftovers from making almond milk
- ½ cup light colored finely grinded flax seed
- ½ cup finely chopped sweet onion
- ¼ cup of virgin olive oil
- 2 crushed cloves of garlic
- 6 fresh finely chopped basil leaves
- 1 teaspoon of Italian seasonings
- A dash Nama Shoyu
- 2 dates
- ½ teaspoon of vanilla essence
- Salt to taste
- Water as needed

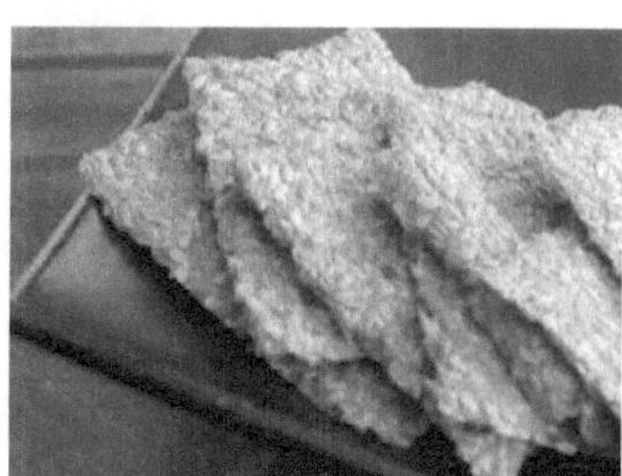

Directions:

1. Soak 1½ cups of almonds in water overnight.
2. Strain and the almonds to the blender with water, dates and vanilla.
3. Blend until very smooth.
4. Strain it however leaving a little moisture in the pulp.
5. Refrigerate the almond milk and use the pulp for the crackers.
6. In a bowl blend all the other ingredients until the mixture is smooth
7. Roll the mixture into small balls on the palm.
8. Place on non-stick dehydrator sheet and press down to shape the cracker.
9. Dehydrate at 105 degrees for 8 hours followed by flipping the crackers over and remove the non-stick sheet.
10. Dehydrate another 6-8 hours until the cracker is dry and crispy.

These crackers can be made in large quantities and can be stored up and eaten along with any raw tea.

Nutty Sour Crumble

Ingredients:

- 1 Cup of Macadamia Nuts

- Zest of Large Lemon

- 4 sticky big Arabic Dates

- 1/4 teaspoon Salt

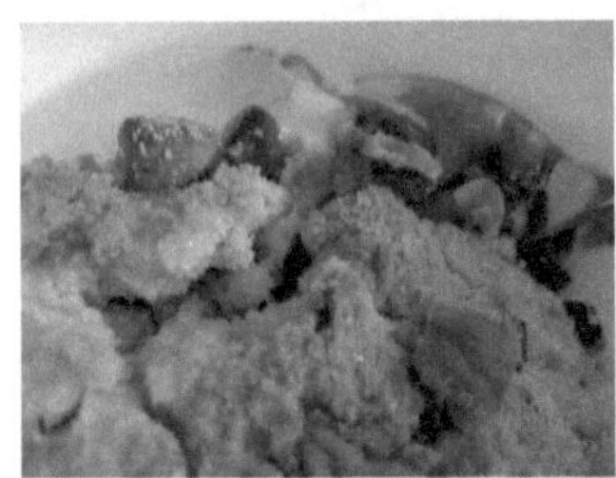

Directions:

It is best to blend the ingredients in a high-speed blender. The crumble will be ready in no time. However, I try and make sure that the ingredients are mixed well but remain chunky. This is pretty quick to prepare and even quicker to eat!

Caramel Chips with Fresh Yoghurt

Ingredients:

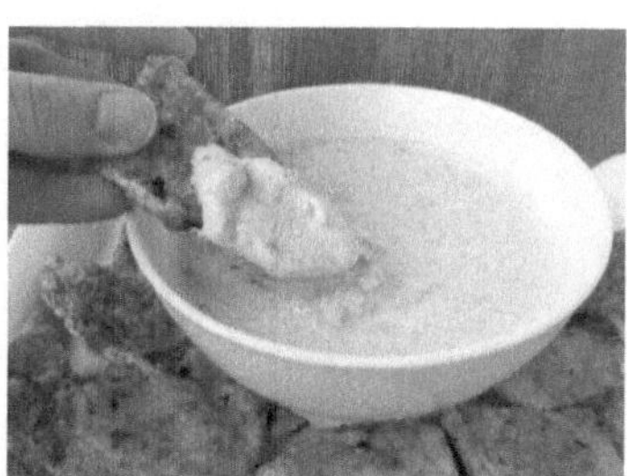

- 1/2 cup soaked cashews (could be soaked for 2-3 hours)

- 1/4 cup of maple syrup

- 1/4 cup of lucuma powder

- 1/2 teaspoon of vanilla extract

- pinch of salt

- Plain Yoghurt

Directions:

1. Blend all the ingredients into a smooth mixture.

2. Place the mixture in a piping bag, with a tip for a shape of your choice and pipe blots onto a dehydrating sheet or tray.

3. Use a dehydrator to heat it at 115 F until its firm for around 12 hours.

4. Store in the refrigerator.

5. In case we don't have a dehydrator, refrigeration could help firm the chips.

Serve it with yoghurt as a delectable and healthy desert. I still enjoy this desert as it is light and is fun yet not too complicated to prepare.

Tropicana Biscotti

Ingredients:

- 1 1/2 cups of almond pulp (leftovers after straining almond milk)

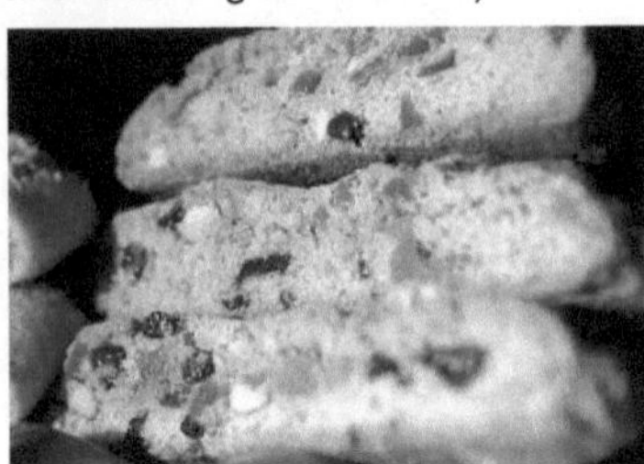

- 1 cup of grounded almonds

- 1 cup of dried Coconut

- 1/2 cup of agave

- 1/2 cup of chopped dried apricots

- 1/2 cup of chopped dried pineapple

- 1/2 cup of currants

- 1 large Orange

Directions:

1. Chop the apricots and pineapple. I normally use a food processor to get it done quickly. Set the chopped fruits aside.

2. Place the cup of almonds in the food processor until we have a smooth residue.

3. Add almond flour and coconut. Blend it in the food processor.

4. Add agave and pulse until a smooth mixture is formed.

5. Place the mixture in a bowl and add orange juice and zest from the orange, but mix it well with hands.

6. Blend in chopped fruit and currants.

7. Form into biscotti shaped loaves and dehydrate 8 hours.

8. Cut it into thinner slices and dehydrate for a few more hours.

9. Store it in the refrigerator.

10.Tastes great with some fat-free cream.

Raw foods dishes are easy to prepare with the help of a dehydrator. They are eco-friendly and even if pregnant mothers are may not go Vegan due to milk being an integral part of their food plan during Pregnancy, a dehydrator makes up for most of the dishes.

Medical and Alternative Solutions for Morning Sickness

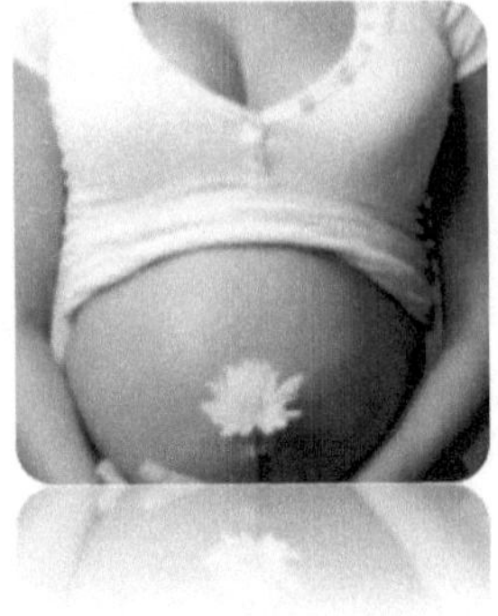

A Quick Overview of Treatments for Morning Sickness

I'll give you a glance over of the most common approaches to morning sickness that exist today.

Medicinal Treatment for Morning Sickness

There are remedies that your physician is likely to prescribe when you complain of morning sickness. These include:

Reflux medicines: Drugs like Pepcid and Zantac are often prescribed for pregnant women if the morning sickness is triggered by reflux.

Droperidol: This is the most commonly prescribed drug for morning sickness, especially for women with hyperemesis gravidarum. Droperidol needs to be administered intravenously, so you will have to be admitted to the hospital for treatment.

Emetrol: This medicine is not formally approved for morning sickness, although it is the only nausea drug that can be bought over the counter.

Compazine, Phenergan and Tigan: These drugs are only available through a prescription. Be careful never to take Compazine and Phenergan at the same time.

Zofran: This medicine is typically used to treat nausea associated with chemotherapy. However, some pregnant women have reported that their nausea is alleviated with this drug. The problem with this drug is that it is quite expensive.

Some of the other medicines that are prescribed as anti-emetics include doxylamine, promethazine, dimenhydrinate, metoclopramide and ondansetron.

The Problem With Using Medical Treatments

Drugs tend to have side effects. The chemicals in the drugs could even affect the baby despite pharmaceutical companies claiming that they don't. Given that the nausea might last for a long time, this does not seem to be the best way to cope with it. It is best to start out by trying natural non-toxic means of reducing the nausea. Only if everything else fails, should one try medicines.

Alternative Treatment for Morning Sickness

Since many women feel very uncomfortable about the idea of using drugs while pregnant, they will feel more attracted to alternative treatments for morning sickness, such as *Acupuncture, Acupressure, Psychology, Hypnosis* and *Aromatherapy* to name a few.
When using an alternative practitioner, always try to either get a referral from a friend who has been treated successfully, or try to find out about the credentials and diploma's of the person you're about to hire.

www.ingramcontent.com/pod-product-compliance
Lightning Source LLC
Chambersburg PA
CBHW031917270726
48655CB00006BA/2337